W9-BYY-655

FRIENDSGIVING

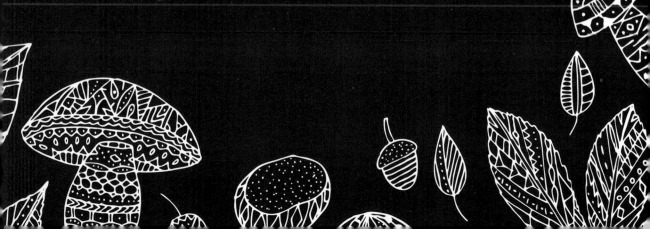

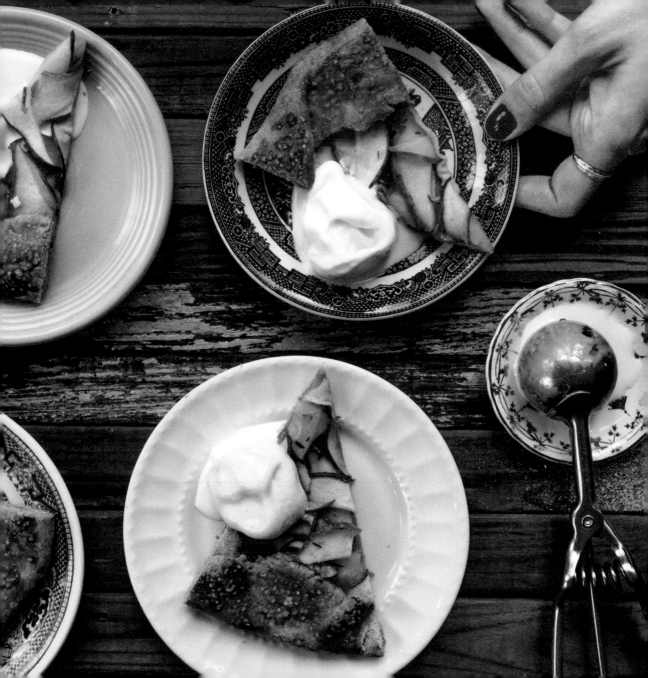

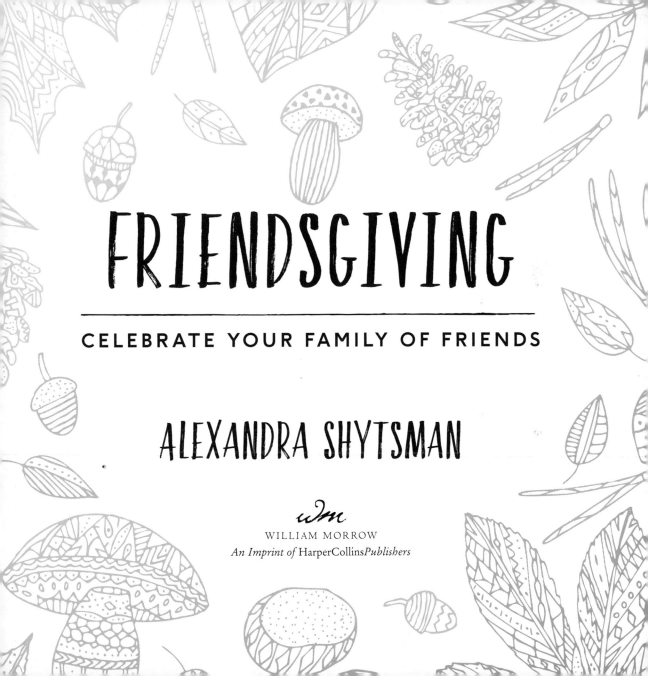

FRIENDSGIVING

CELEBRATE YOUR FAMILY OF FRIENDS

ALEXANDRA SHYTSMAN

WM
WILLIAM MORROW
An Imprint of HarperCollins*Publishers*

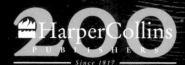

FRIENDSGIVING. Copyright © 2017 by Alexandra Shytsman. All rights reserved. Printed in the United States of America. No part of this book may be used or reproduced in any manner whatsoever without written permission except in the case of brief quotations embodied in critical articles and reviews. For information address HarperCollins Publishers, 195 Broadway, New York, NY 10007.

HarperCollins books may be purchased for educational, business, or sales promotional use. For information please e-mail the Special Markets Department at SPsales@harpercollins.com.

FIRST EDITION

Designed by Suet Yee Chong
Illustrations by Anastasia Panfilova/Shutterstock, Inc.
Photography by Alexandra Shytsman
Food and prop styling by Alexandra Shytsman and Rebecca Ffrench
Food styling assisting by Sean Arguelles
Author photograph by Michelle Fidman

Library of Congress Cataloging-in-Publication Data has been applied for.

ISBN 978-0-06-269819-3

17 18 19 20 21   LSC   10 9 8 7 6 5 4 3 2 1

To my mom,
for teaching me the importance of home cooking
and the joy of gathering around a table.

And to all the wonderful people
I am lucky to call my friends.

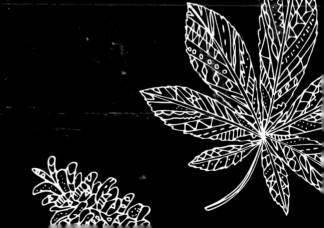

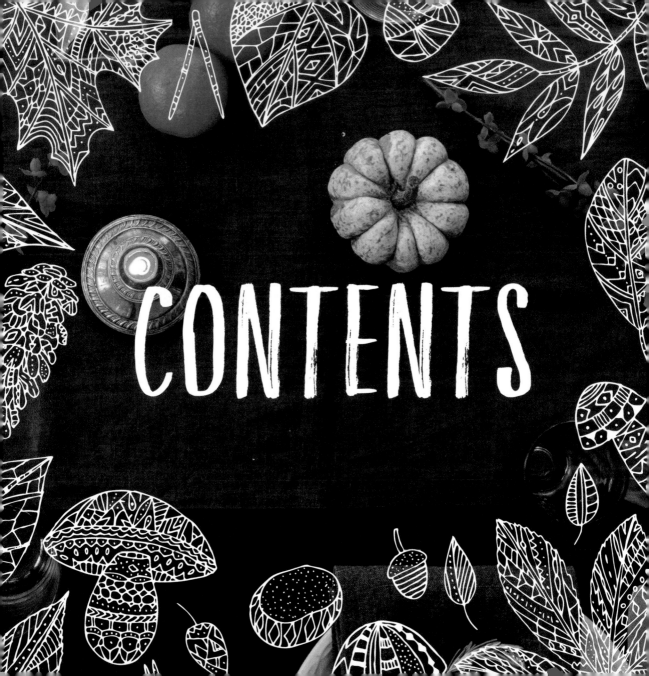

CONTENTS

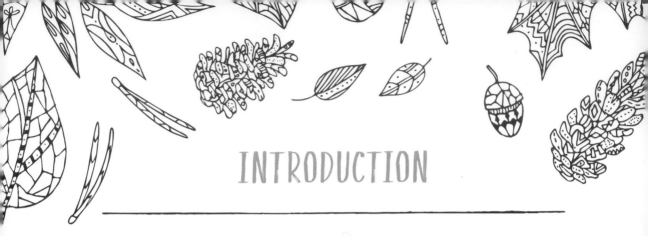

INTRODUCTION

Friendsgiving is my favorite holiday of the year—albeit a made-up one. Friendsgiving is everything you love about Thanksgiving—hearty food, day drinking, good company—without the things you don't love, like nagging family members and heated political discussions that make you question if maybe you were adopted after all . . .

Friendsgiving is a special tradition for me. As Ukrainian immigrants, my family and I did not always celebrate Thanksgiving. When my sister and I were in high school, my parents would hang out with their fellow immigrant friends on Thanksgiving Day (since everyone had the day off), leaving us home alone. Like any parent-free high schoolers on a federal holiday, we threw parties. But they weren't your average house parties—they were dinner parties where I first got to try my hand at cooking American Thanksgiving food. (Of course, Friendsgiving was the second dinner most of my friends were attending, but they made sure to save room.)

In the weeks leading up to my first Friendsgiving, I obsessively watched every single Thanksgiving special on the Food Network, where I learned how to combat a dry turkey and to make something so seemingly silly as stuffing (I mean, it's basically old bread revived with some veggies and stock) actually taste good. I'll never forget the feeling of triumph when I pulled my first turkey out of the oven and proceeded to carve it as I'd seen done on TV. I was as surprised as anyone to learn that it was in fact cooked through, juicy, and delicious. Another dish that appeared on my first Friendsgiving table was caramelized onion and goat cheese crostini. I don't recall where the idea initially came from, but I do remember my friends helping me assemble them as I was putting the final touches on the main meal, which ultimately became the inspiration for my Choose-Your-Own-Adventure Crostini Bar (page 19).

Sure, back then we may have eaten off paper plates and had Jell-O shots for dessert, but I assure you my Friendsgivings were the most grown-up high-school parties in all of South Brooklyn. The tradition continued well into our college years and beyond, as there is no better way to usher in the festive spirit of the holidays than gathering your favorite people at home for a cozy meal. Each year I look forward to adding new dishes and flavors to the menu, and watching my friends' excitement as they approach the dinner table. (We've also graduated from paper plates to ceramic, thank you very much.)

Thus, I am thrilled to share my passion for hosting a proper Friendsgiving with you in this compact volume. I hope that as you make your way through this book, you'll be inspired to start a Friendsgiving tradition of your own.

HAPPY FRIENDSGIVING!

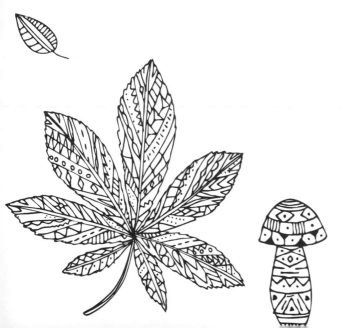

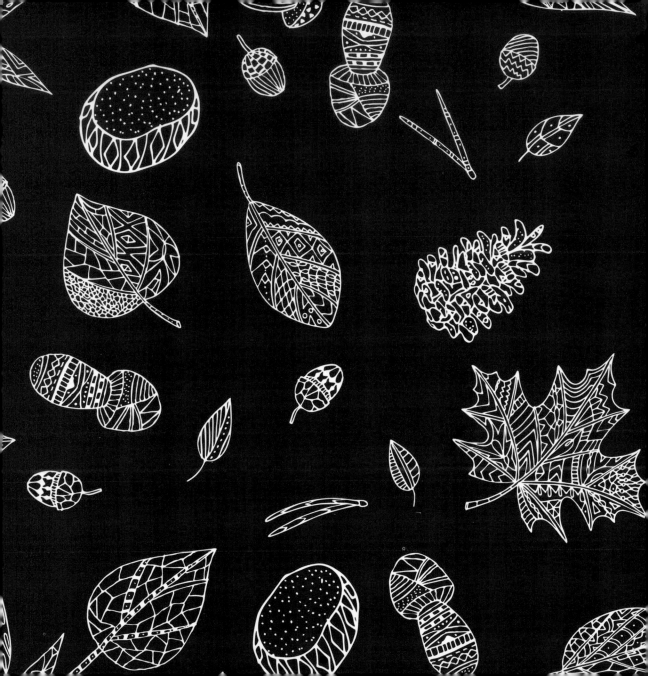

SO YOU'RE HOSTING FRIENDSGIVING... NOW WHAT?

TIPS FOR USING THIS BOOK

This book consists of five themed dinner menus, a handful of appetizer ideas that can be mixed and matched, and three desserts that pair well with all the menus.

If you're having a smaller gathering, prepare either the Choose-Your-Own-Adventure Crostini Bar (page 19) or the two dips (see page 24) from the Pregame chapter, and pair it with just one cocktail (see pages 28 and 29). If you're having a larger group, feel free to make as many appetizers and drinks as you like.

Each of the themed menus in this book is designed to create a unique Friendsgiving party. If you're a purist, go for the turkey-centric Classic menu (page 31). But since Friendsgiving is typically a more casual affair (and Aunt Marge is not there to yell at you about how things are "supposed to be"), the three menus that follow are inspired by my favorite global flavors and feature dishes that are perfect for sharing with friends. You'll notice that the last menu, the Modern (page 79), is a take on a sophisticated vegan, gluten-free meal. With so many people adopting healthier lifestyles these days, I wanted to make sure there's something in this book for everyone. All five of the menus are scaled to feed six to eight guests family-style and list the recipes in the order they should be cooked.

Want to go rogue and design your own dinner menu? No problem—choose your favorite recipe from each section and go to town. For instance, there's no reason why the turkey from the Classic menu can't be served with the chickpea-celeriac puree from the Modern menu, the fried chicken from the Southern menu with the kale and butternut squash salad from the Italian menu, and so forth.

Want to host Friendsgiving in June? That's cool, too! These recipes are versatile enough to adapt to any season or type of party.

As for dessert, two are always better than one. I always recommend serving some kind of pie or fruit tart, like my Pear-Thyme Whole Wheat Galette (page 91)—it's harvest season after all!—paired with another crowd-pleasing sweet treat. Check out the Spicy Dark Chocolate Bark with Cranberries, Hazelnuts, and Sea Salt (page 96), the Vegan Autumn-Spice Panna Cotta (page 93), or pick up some store-bought cookies and pastries.

Freaking out about hosting your first Friendsgiving? Take a deep breath and flip to page 12, where you'll find the aptly named "Timeline to Get It All Done." This breakdown will guide you through the whole enchilada—starting from two weeks out and taking you through that last hour before your friends arrive. Each menu has its own timeline, too, so you'll know exactly when to chop, blend, and sauté all the things.

At the beginning of each menu, you'll also find tips titled "A Little Help from Your Friends," which include answers to the inevitable "Can I bring anything?" question you'll be asked. And if wine is the specific contribution you prefer, there are suggestions for that, too.

DISCLAIMER: If you are familiar with my blog, *The New Baguette,* you know that I am an advocate for plant-centric eating most of the time. However, I do believe there are times for indulging in celebration food, and Friendsgiving is definitely one of them. With that said, I urge you to pay close attention to the quality of your ingredients, using, whenever possible, local organic produce and pasture-raised, grass-fed animal proteins that were grown without hormones or antibiotics. While it may be a little pricier, it's a worthy investment for your health and that of the planet.

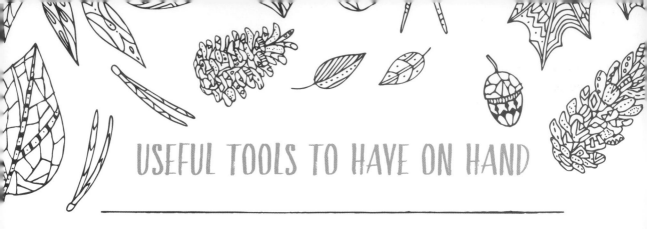

USEFUL TOOLS TO HAVE ON HAND

CHEF'S KNIFE: A professional chef's knife is the best gift you can give yourself as a home cook. There is no need for that bulky knife set that sits on your counter and collects dust. Owning just one good knife will cut your prep time in half and come in handy (puns intended) for the toughest of jobs—like carving the turkey (see page 34), peeling yuca (see page 50), or dissecting a butternut squash (see page 71). I've used the same Mercer brand 8-inch chef's knife for the past ten years.

LARGE CUTTING BOARD: Your board should be large enough for you to comfortably use both your hands as you chop, freely rocking your knife back and forth, and to allow you to chop a decent amount of produce without having to clear off the board before chopping more. To keep your board from sliding as you chop, anchor it by placing a wet paper towel underneath it.

MEASURING CUPS AND SPOONS: Using proper ingredient amounts is a key contributor to the success of a recipe, especially when it comes to dessert.

FOOD PROCESSOR: A food processor is the single most important small kitchen appliance. It makes dips, spreads, purees, pesto, and pie crusts, and those are just the recipes included in this book.

MEAT THERMOMETER: If you get nervous about eating undercooked animal proteins, using an instant-read meat thermometer will alleviate your worries. If you're cooking turkey, it's especially important to make sure you reach the right internal temperature (165°F).

OTHER KITCHEN TOOLS: One or two large nonstick skillets, one or two standard rimmed baking sheets, a couple of pots, and a Dutch oven or high-sided roasting pan will all make cooking for a dinner party a breeze.

PARTY ESSENTIALS

For the day of the party, be sure to have bags of ice, extra drinking cups, a wine bottle opener, and cocktail napkins.

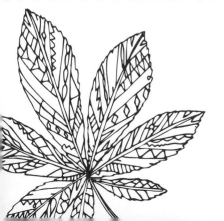

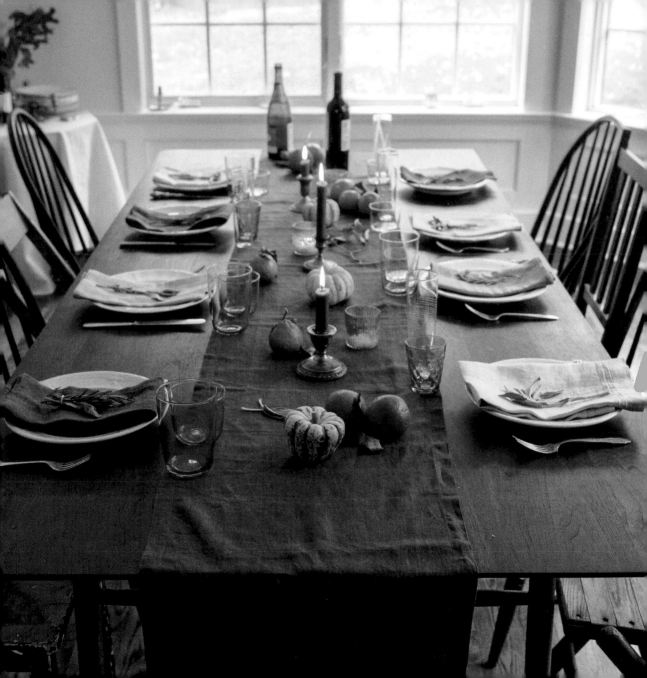

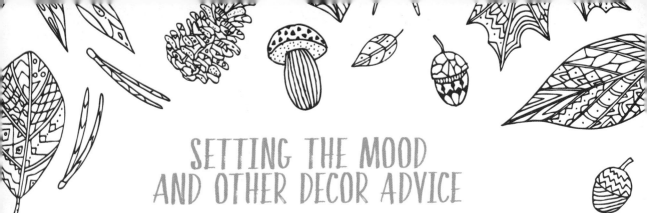

SETTING THE MOOD AND OTHER DECOR ADVICE

Although hanging banners, strewing about mini gourds, or arranging seasonal flowers is nice, it's not always necessary. The main objective is to create a cozy environment, so start by setting the mood:

- Tidy up and eliminate clutter wherever possible.

- Make sure there are enough comfy spots for people to hang out (a few floor cushions and throw blankets can go a long way).

- Dim the lights and light candles.

- Play some tunes (try my favorite playlist on page 108).

Once your home or apartment is party ready, you can add in the extra bits of festive decor (if desired). Here's how to get the ultimate Friendsgiving look:

- Pick up a few varieties of yellow-and-orange-hued flowers, mix and match them to make a couple of floral arrangements, and place them around your home.

- Use a dark blue or purple table runner to complement the yellow and orange hues.

7

- Hang a Happy Thanksgiving banner, festive garlands, or string lights.

- Print out "I'm thankful for . . ." cards for your friends to fill out (find a design online or create your own)—these will make great party favors.

CENTERPIECE IDEAS

Elements of nature are the perfect way to dress up your Friendsgiving table. Think small winter squashes, bowls of citrus fruit, apples, or pears, and bundles of hardy herbs like rosemary, sage, and thyme. Not only beautiful, but they're also widely available, affordable, and you can eat them afterward! If you choose to put candles on the table, make sure they are unscented—you don't want anything interfering with the delicious meal you've prepared.

PLACE SETTINGS

I prefer not to assign seats at dinner parties, as I find that most people gravitate toward certain places. However, to dress up each place setting, I like to use a sprig of rosemary, sage, or thyme atop a folded napkin. You can also use mini pumpkins (even spray-paint them gold, if you like!), mandarin oranges, or pinecones—just make sure you clean them first.

NO DINING TABLE? NO PROBLEM

Set up a buffet on your kitchen counter or coffee table (if it's large enough), and gather in the living room—your friends won't mind one bit eating off their laps. Just make sure there

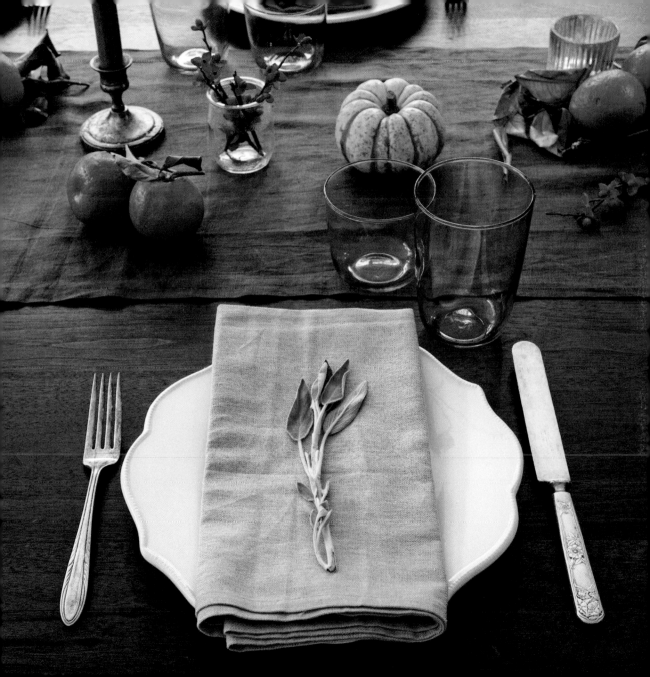

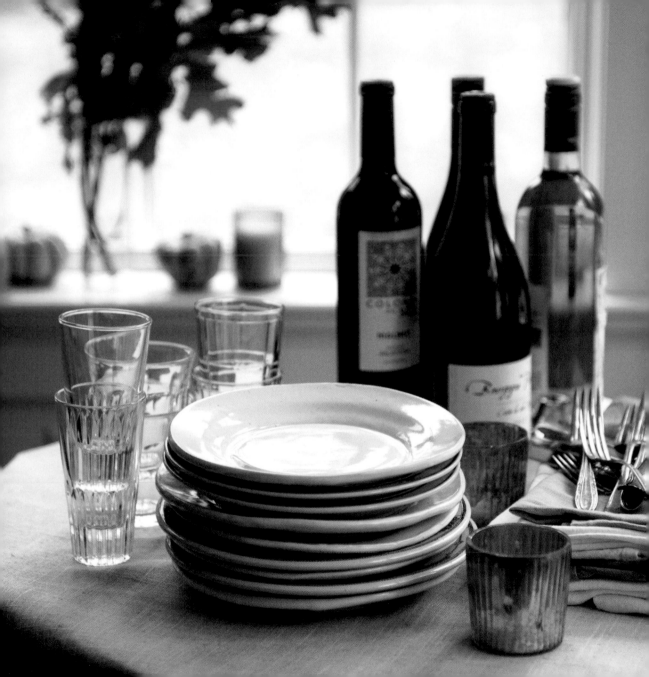

is enough room for people to set down their drinks. Need an extra surface? You can buy an IKEA side table for around $15.

A WORD ON DINNERWARE

When hosting one to eight guests, use real plates, glasses, silverware, and so on (it does not have to be a matching set). Eight or more? Disposable is fine. Just make sure it's the nice stuff—no paper or styrofoam on the best faux-holiday of the year. And be sure to recycle afterward. Alternatively, these days lots of companies are making biodegradable options from natural materials, like fallen leaves (yes, really) and sugarcane, which are not only environmentally friendly but beautiful, too. If you're over the age of twenty-one, those big red plastic cups are so not okay. Opt for small clear tumblers instead.

A NOTE ON WINE

The golden rule of serving wine at a party is that guests usually drink about two glasses per hour. One 750 mL bottle of wine yields six 4-ounce glasses. So if you have eight guests and your dinner lasts about two hours, you will need thirty-two glasses of wine—about five bottles.

It's a good idea to also have some beer on hand—just nothing too heavy, like porters or stouts. Cider goes well with Friendsgiving, too, but steer clear of anything too sweet.

TIMELINE TO GET IT ALL DONE

2 WEEKS IN ADVANCE . . .

Plan your menu.

Send out the e-invitation.

Assess your space (need extra tables, chairs, silverware, etc.?) and make necessary arrangements.

1 WEEK IN ADVANCE . . .

Buy grocery staples (dry and boxed goods).

Assign items for your friends to bring.

3 DAYS IN ADVANCE . . .

Move your turkey (if serving) from freezer to fridge.

2 DAYS IN ADVANCE . . .

Buy the fresh produce and animal proteins.

Tidy up your space and decorate (if desired).

THE DAY BEFORE . . .

Buy ice (if needed).

Dry-brine your turkey (if serving).

Complete basic prep where possible (soak beans, clean and chop vegetables, make galette dough, etc.)—be sure to read through your recipes to assess prep and cook times, and check for "Do Ahead" sections below each recipe.

THE DAY OF . . .

Wake up at a decent hour.

Shower and get ready early: I like to get this over with before I start cooking so I'm not rushing when guests arrive.

Chill wine and beer (if serving).

Set the table.

Make a Friendsgiving meal!

AN HOUR BEFORE GUESTS ARRIVE . . .

Make final preparations: clean up the the kitchen, call friends to request last-minute items.

Change into your party outfit.

A FEW MINUTES BEFORE . . .

Put out the pregame snacks and drinks.

Pour yourself a drink (you deserve it).

Turn on the tunes and greet your guests!

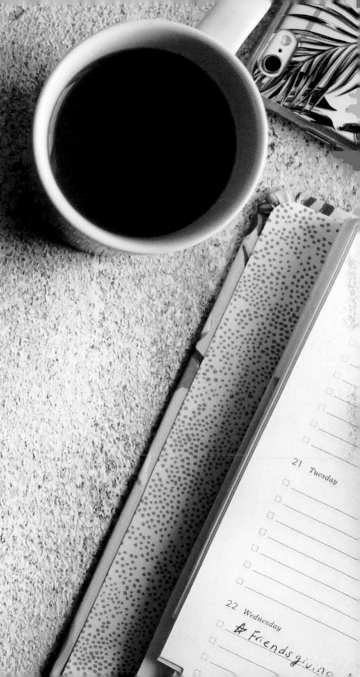

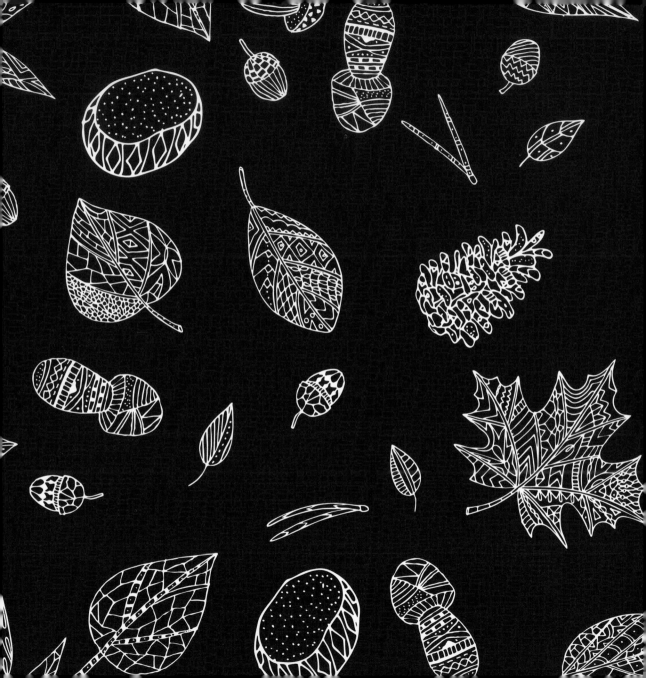

MENUS

+

RECIPES

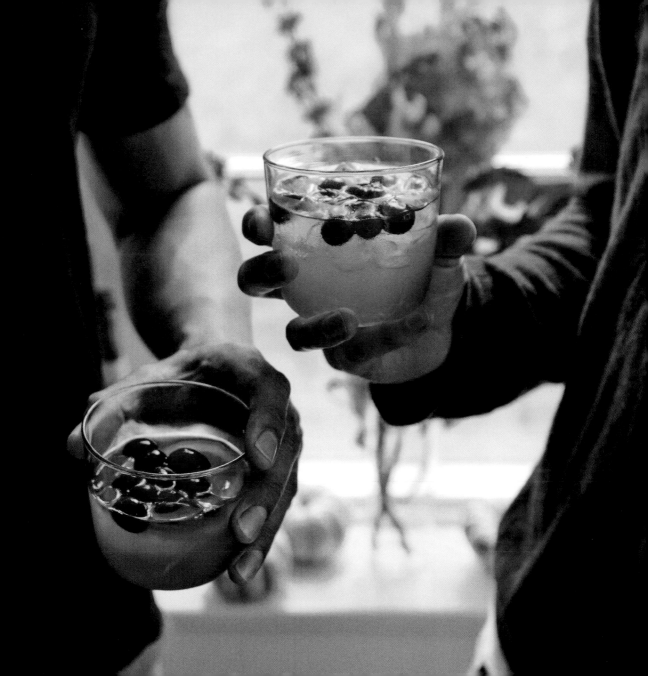

PREGAME

It's imperative to have some snacks and drinks ready to go when people walk in the door. Want to turn cocktail hour into an activity? Set up a crostini bar and let your friends do the mixing and matching. Got friends on the lazier side? Make the two dips instead.

Choose-Your-Own-Adventure Crostini Bar
19

Muhammara
24

Sweet Potato–Tahini Dip with Za'atar
25

Earl Grey–Ginger Rum Punch
28

Lillet Blanc–Cassis Spritzer
29

A LITTLE HELP FROM YOUR FRIENDS
Gourmet condiments (think flavored mustard and aged balsamic vinegar), fancy crackers, and spiced nuts are just a few of the items you can ask for.

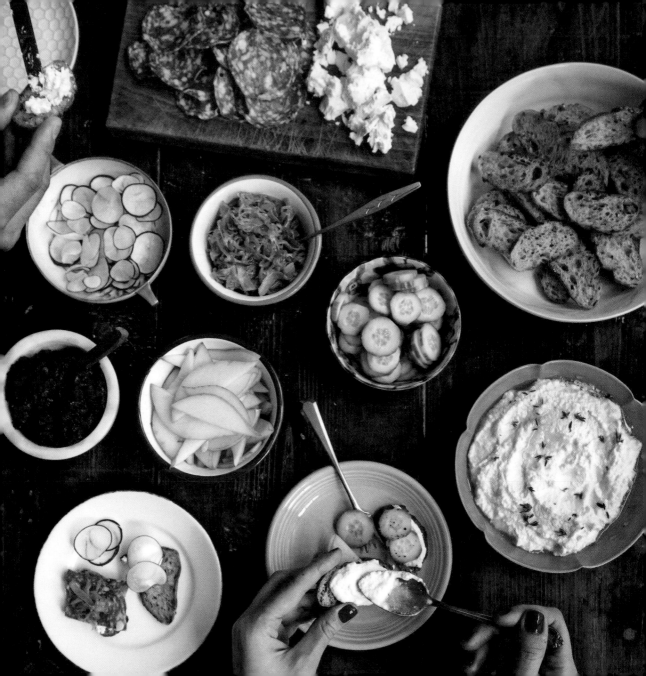

CHOOSE-YOUR-OWN-ADVENTURE CROSTINI BAR

A DIY crostini bar is awesome for several reasons:

- It keeps people out of the kitchen, allowing you to put final touches on things without distractions.

- It's a good icebreaker if you have guests who are meeting each other for the first time.

- It helps guests feel that they participated in the preparation of the meal.

I love to make caramelized onions and sun-dried tomato tapenade from scratch and supplement the bar spread with various toppings. I like to use sliced vegetables and fruits—like radishes, cucumbers, and pears—along with cured meats, crumbled goat cheese, and ricotta drizzled with honey and thyme.

TO MAKE CROSTINI

Preheat the oven to 375°F. Slice a baguette into thin rounds, place them on a baking sheet in a single layer, and drizzle lightly with olive oil. Bake until crisp and golden brown, about 10 minutes.

TO MAKE CARAMELIZED ONIONS

Heat **1 tablespoon olive oil** and **1 tablespoon butter** in a large heavy-bottomed skillet over low heat. Add **4 small thinly sliced yellow onions**, **½ teaspoon salt**, and toss to coat in the oil. Cover tightly with a lid and cook until the steam has softened the onions and they start to become translucent, stirring occasionally, about 7 minutes. Remove the lid and increase the heat to medium-low. Stir in **¾ teaspoon dried thyme** and ¼ **teaspoon freshly ground black pepper.** Cook until onions are caramel-colored and pasty, stirring frequently, about 25 minutes.

TO MAKE SUN-DRIED TOMATO TAPENADE

In a food processor, combine **1 cup pitted and rinsed Kalamata olives** with **1 cup sun-dried tomatoes** jarred in oil and drained. Pulse until broken down. Add **2 tablespoons drained capers, 1 teaspoon herbes de Provence, 1 medium garlic clove,** and ¼ **teaspoon freshly ground black pepper** and pulse to combine.

FRIENDSGIVING PRO TIP

You may be the host, but you don't have to do everything yourself. Both of these crostini toppings are easy enough for anyone to handle, and because they travel well and can be served at room temperature, ask a friend to bring them.

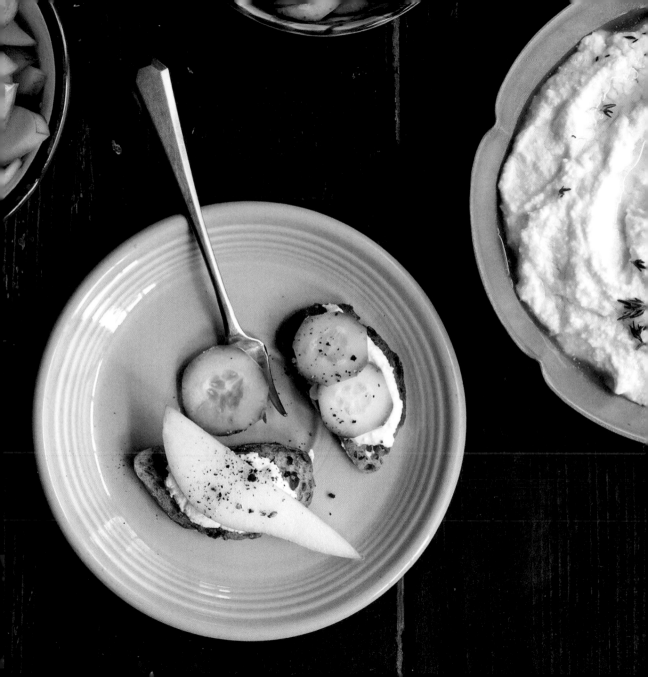

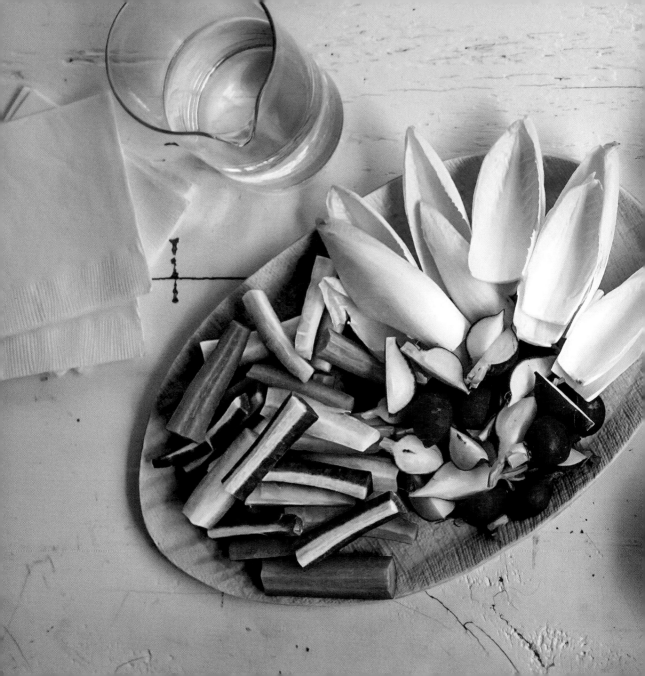

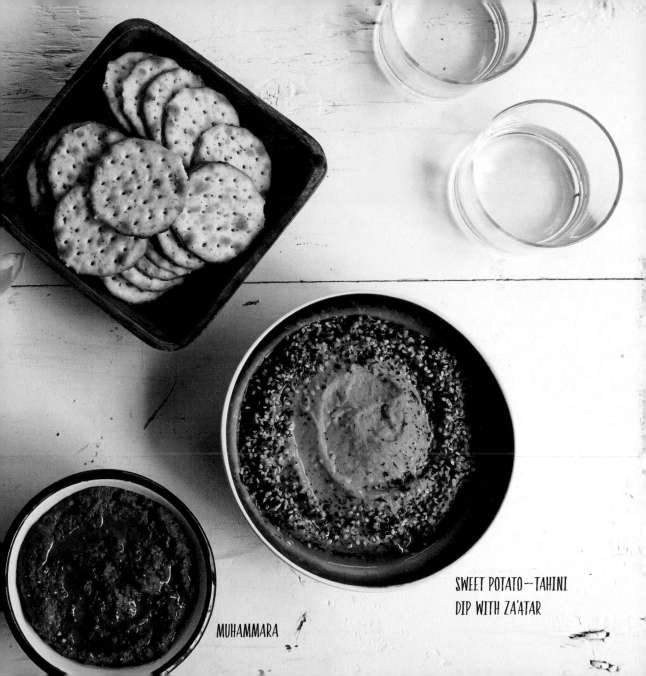

MUHAMMARA

SWEET POTATO—TAHINI
DIP WITH ZA'ATAR

MUHAMMARA

Muhammara is a traditional Syrian spread. It's awesome as a dip or as a condiment for cooked vegetables and grilled meats. *Muhammara* is typically made with pomegranate molasses, but since it can be hard to find, I use reduced balsamic vinegar for a similar result. If you do locate the molasses, feel free to use 2 teaspoon of that instead—no need to reduce it, though.

¼ cup balsamic vinegar

1 cup jarred roasted red peppers, drained

½ cup walnuts, toasted

2 small garlic cloves, roughly chopped

2 tablespoons freshly squeezed lemon juice (from about 1 lemon)

1 teaspoon ground cumin

Pinch of ground cayenne pepper

¼ cup extra-virgin olive oil

Sea salt and freshly ground black pepper

1. Pour the vinegar into a small saucepan and bring to a boil. Reduce the heat to a bare simmer and cook until thick and syrupy, 3 to 4 minutes.

2. In a food processor, combine the red peppers, walnuts, bread crumbs, garlic, lemon juice, cumin, cayenne, and 2 teaspoons of the reduced vinegar. Pulse until the mixture begins to come together. With the motor running, slowly stream in the oil through the chute of the food processor and puree until the mixture comes together but is still a bit chunky. Season to taste with salt and pepper, or more lemon juice, if needed.

3. Serve with crudités, crackers, and/or pita chips.

SWEET POTATO–TAHINI DIP WITH ZA'ATAR

MAKES ABOUT 2 CUPS (SERVES 8 AS AN APPETIZER)

Since the base of this dip is so simple—it's mostly sweet potatoes and tahini—homemade *za'atar* (a Middle Eastern spice blend) really helps the flavors stand out. This recipe makes a bit more *za'atar* than you'll actually need, so use the leftovers to sprinkle on roasted vegetables or on bread dipped in olive oil.

2 small sweet potatoes (about 1 pound), scrubbed

1 tablespoon raw sesame seeds

1 tablespoon minced fresh thyme

1 tablespoon sumac

Coarse sea salt

2 tablespoons tahini

2 tablespoons filtered water

1 tablespoon freshly squeezed lemon juice (from about ½ lemon)

A few dashes of your favorite hot sauce

Freshly ground black pepper

1 teaspoon extra-virgin olive oil

1. Preheat the oven to 400°F.

2. Pierce the sweet potatoes all over with a fork and wrap each one tightly in foil. Place on a baking sheet and roast until the flesh gives easily when pressed, about 1 hour. Unwrap and set aside to cool completely.

3. To make the *za'atar*, toast the sesame seeds in a small skillet over low heat until golden and fragrant, about 3 minutes. Transfer to a bowl and add the thyme, sumac, and ¼ teaspoon salt. Stir and set aside.

4. Peel the sweet potatoes and place them in a food processor. Add the tahini, water, lemon juice, hot sauce, a few turns of pepper, and 2 teaspoons of the prepared *za'atar*. Puree until completely smooth. Taste and season with more salt and pepper, if needed.

5. Scrape the dip into a small serving bowl, drizzle with the oil, and sprinkle with a teaspoon of the *za'atar*.

DO AHEAD: *Both dips can be made up to a day in advance and stored in airtight containers in the fridge.*

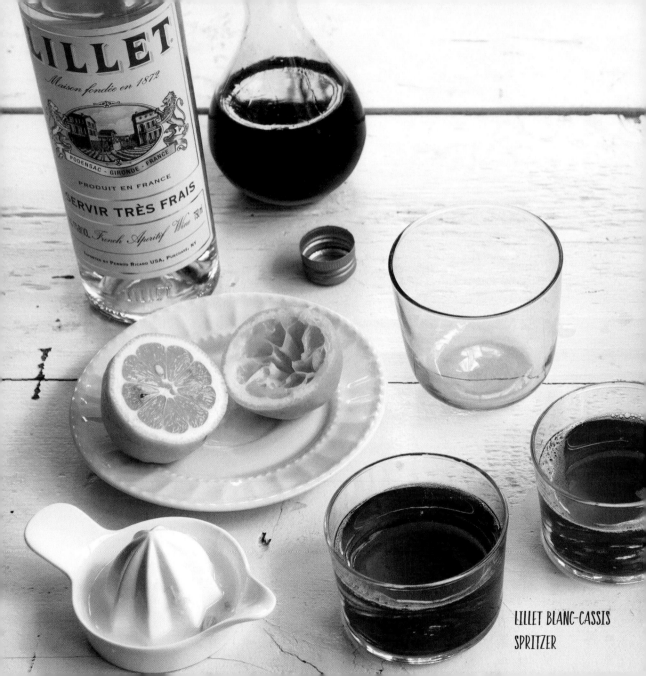

LILLET BLANC-CASSIS
SPRITZER

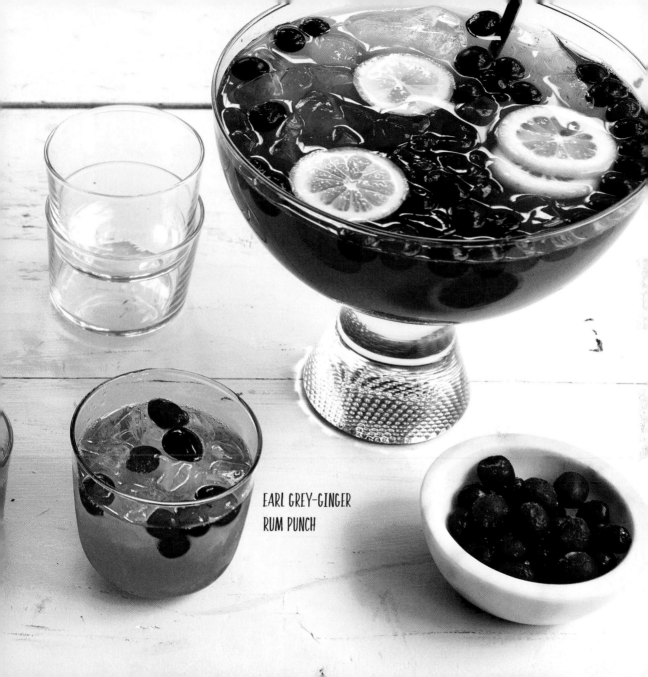

EARL GREY-GINGER
RUM PUNCH

EARL GREY–GINGER RUM PUNCH

MAKES 8 DRINKS

You know that wide-eyed look that spreads across your friends' faces when a pitcher of sangria approaches your table at a restaurant? That is exactly the type of enthusiasm you want to infuse into your Friendsgiving. Punch bowl and pitcher cocktails allow you to make big batches of drinks instead of mixing each one individually every time someone is thirsty. (Read: less work, more party).
I love how Earl Grey's bitterness and the bergamot aroma pair with warming rum. The ginger beer adds a kick of fall spice, and the cranberries brighten up the combination.

---

4 cups boiling water

2 bags Earl Grey tea

1 tablespoon plus 1 teaspoon honey

Ice

1 cup gold rum

One 16-ounce bottle ginger beer

Lemon wheels and frozen cranberries, for garnish

1. In a heat-proof container, combine the water and tea bags and let steep for 10 minutes. Discard the tea bags and stir the honey into the tea until fully dissolved. Chill until completely cool.

2. Transfer the tea to a punch bowl or pitcher, and add the ice, rum, and ginger beer. Stir to combine and garnish with lemon wheels and cranberries.

DO AHEAD: *The tea may be steeped up to a day in advance and stored in an airtight container in the fridge.*

LILLET BLANC—CASSIS SPRITZER

Lillet is a French fortified wine that's typically consumed as an aperitif over ice with an orange twist. It comes in white, red, and rosé varieties—the white being the most popular. (Fact: Lillet is my most favorite drink; if you're ever invited over to my place, bring a bottle of this stuff and we'll be friends forever.) Cassis—a sweet, syrupy black currant liqueur—also comes from France, specifically the eponymous region near Marseille.
This drink is sweet, fruity, and perfect for the holidays!

Combine **2 cups Lillet Blanc** and **½ cup crème de cassis** in a pitcher. Top with **2 cups chilled dry sparkling wine**. Serve immediately.

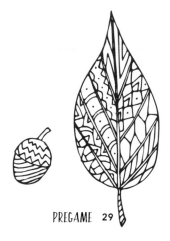

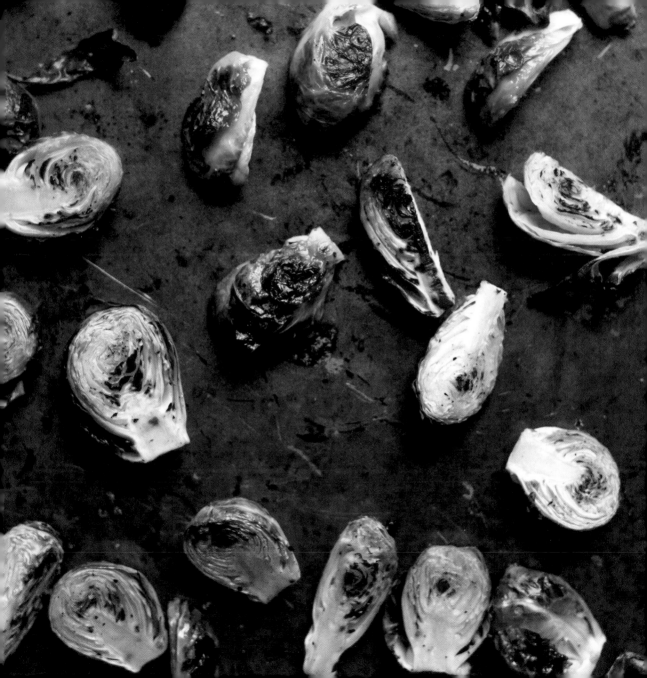

THE CLASSIC

Is Friendsgiving the only Thanksgiving meal you're having this year? Here's the traditional turkey-centric menu you need.

Dry-Brined Roasted Turkey
with Gravy
33

Charred Balsamic Brussels Sprouts
with Feta and Pomegranate Seeds
39

Stuffing with Italian Sausage and
Caramelized Fennel
36

Sour Cream Smashed Potatoes
with Fried Shallots
41

TIMELINE

1 DAY AHEAD: Dry-brine the turkey.

4 TO 5 HOURS AHEAD: Start roasting the turkey.

2 HOURS AHEAD: Make the stuffing.

1 HOUR AHEAD: Make the Brussels sprouts and potatoes, then the gravy.

A LITTLE HELP FROM YOUR FRIENDS

A classic menu calls for classic dishes. Ask friends to bring dinner rolls, cranberry sauce, and a sweet potato pie.

SUGGESTED WINE PAIRINGS

Sauvignon Blanc, Chardonnay, or Beaujolais Nouveau

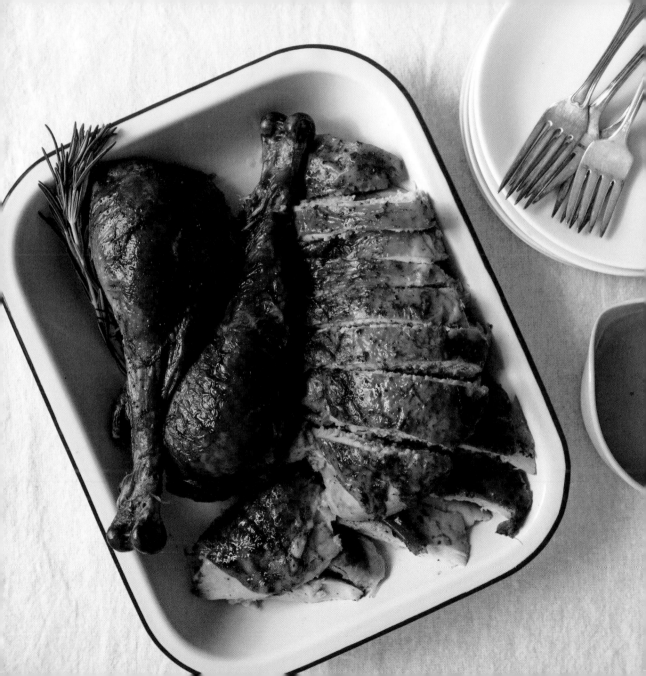

DRY-BRINED ROASTED TURKEY WITH GRAVY

If this is your first time roasting a turkey, the most important thing is not to panic. Just think of it as a big chicken. You are the boss of this bird, and I know you can do it. There are just a few key things to remember. First, use a dry brine, which is just a fancy way of saying seasoning the turkey one day in advance and letting the salt do its magic. Second, use plenty of aromatics to flavor the bird. Third, you gotta baste that thing like it's your job. And last, let the turkey rest before carving it (see step 7) to keep it juicy inside.

SPECIAL EQUIPMENT

Kitchen twine and meat thermometer

TURKEY

One 12- to 14-pound turkey, fully thawed if frozen

Sea salt and freshly ground black pepper

1 tablespoon unsalted butter

1 tablespoon extra-virgin olive oil

1 teaspoon poultry seasoning

2 fresh rosemary or thyme sprigs or one of each

continues on next page

1. To brine the turkey: Check the neck and body cavities of the turkey, and discard any packaging and bag of giblets. Pat the turkey completely dry with paper towels. Generously season the turkey with salt and pepper, making sure to massage all over, including under the skin. Place the turkey into any container large enough to hold it (like a stockpot or a roasting pan) and cover loosely with foil. Refrigerate overnight.

2. To roast the turkey: Position the oven rack to the lowest third of the oven. Preheat the oven to 400°F.

3. Combine the butter, oil, and poultry seasoning in a small saucepan over medium-low heat until the butter is melted and bubbly; set aside.

4. Place the turkey into a roasting pan and tuck the wings under. Stuff the turkey with the herbs, lemon, onion, and garlic—as much as will fit in the body cavity; scatter the

1 lemon, cut into wedges

1 small yellow onion, roughly chopped

4 garlic cloves, smashed and roughly chopped

2 cups low-sodium turkey or chicken stock

GRAVY

2 tablespoons extra-virgin olive oil

2 tablespoons all-purpose flour

3 cups reserved turkey cooking liquid

rest in the roasting pan around the turkey. Using kitchen twine, tie the legs together.

5. Pour the butter-olive oil mixture over the turkey and massage it to coat the turkey evenly. Pour the stock into the roasting pan and cover the turkey loosely with foil. Roast for 45 minutes.

6. Reduce the oven temperature to 350°F and uncover the turkey. Roast for 30 minutes, then begin to baste the turkey in its stock, either using a baster or a small ladle. Continue roasting the turkey until an oven thermometer inserted into the thickest part of the thigh reaches 165°F, about 3 hours, basting the turkey every 30 minutes until it is cooked.

7. Remove the turkey from the oven and let it rest for about 10 minutes, until it stops steaming. Transfer the turkey to a baking sheet, being careful not to tear the skin. Discard the herbs and vegetables left over in the roasting pan, and reserve 3 cups of the cooking liquid. Cover the turkey loosely with foil and let stand for 30 minutes.

8. Meanwhile, make the gravy: Strain the turkey cooking liquid and discard the solids. Heat the oil over medium-low heat in a medium saucepan. Whisk in the flour and cook for 1 minute. Whisk in the cooking liquid and bring to a boil. Reduce the heat to low and simmer until thickened, about 8 minutes, whisking frequently.

9. Carve the turkey: Be sure to use a sharp knife! Starting with the legs, cut into where the leg meets the body

until you hit the joint, then slice through the joint to separate the leg. Repeat on the other side. To carve the breast, make one long cut into one side of the breast alongside the breastbone, then position your knife near the underside of the turkey and slice until you reach the initial slit. Place the breast meat on a cutting board and repeat on the other side. Slice both breasts into 1-inch slices and serve alongside the gravy.

FRIENDSGIVING PRO TIP

The basic rule of serving turkey at a dinner party is 1 pound per person. I always size up, since I love cooking with leftover turkey. Alternatively, in classic eastern European fashion, send guests home with leftovers so they can enjoy a turkey sandwich for breakfast the next day.

LEFTOVER STRATEGY

Make turkey noodle soup! Sauté onions, carrots, and celery in a heavy-bottomed pot until softened. Add leftover turkey legs, wings, bones, and stock or water. Bring to a boil, then simmer for 20 minutes. Add leftover shredded white meat and egg noodles. Simmer for a few minutes, until the noodles are tender. Garnish with chopped fresh parsley.

STUFFING WITH ITALIAN SAUSAGE AND CARAMELIZED FENNEL

It's definitely best to make stuffing in a separate casserole dish rather than stuffed inside the turkey; it's safer, since bacteria from the turkey drippings are not entirely sanitary, and you'd also end up with really soggy stuffing. I love the way this stuffing has a soft, pillowy interior with a crunchy top.

1 loaf of white Italian bread, cut into ½-inch cubes (9 to 10 cups)

About 3 tablespoons extra-virgin olive oil

2 spicy Italian sausages, casings removed

1 medium yellow onion, finely diced

1 large carrot, finely diced

1 teaspoon poultry seasoning

Sea salt and freshly ground black pepper

1 large garlic clove, minced

1 large fennel bulb, quartered, cored, and thinly sliced

1. Preheat the oven to 350°F.

2. Place the bread cubes on a baking sheet and bake until dried out and lightly toasted, about 12 minutes; set aside.

3. Heat 1 teaspoon of the oil in a large nonstick skillet over medium-high heat. Add the sausage meat and cook until it is evenly browned, breaking it up with a wooden spatula, 5 to 7 minutes. Transfer to a small bowl and set aside. Reserve the remaining fat in the skillet.

4. Return the skillet to medium-low heat and add about 2 teaspoons of the oil, so there is enough fat to coat the bottom. Add the onion, carrot, poultry seasoning, and ¼ teaspoon of both salt and pepper. Cook until the vegetables are softened, stirring occasionally, about 10 minutes. Add the garlic and cook for another minute.

5. Meanwhile, heat 2 tablespoons of the oil in a separate large skillet over high heat and add the fennel. Cook,

2½ cups low-sodium chicken or turkey stock

1 tablespoon unsalted butter, melted

stirring occasionally, until the fennel is nicely browned, about 12 minutes.

6. Lightly grease a 9 × 13-inch baking dish with oil and set aside.

7. In a large bowl, combine the croutons, sausage, onion-carrot mixture, and fennel (if you don't have a large enough bowl, do this in batches). Gradually stir in the stock to ensure the croutons are evenly hydrated. Transfer the mixture to the prepared baking dish and drizzle with the butter. Bake until golden brown, about 20 minutes.

NOTE: *In a pinch, feel free to buy bagged croutons, which are usually available in supermarkets this time of year—just make sure they're not flavored.*

DO AHEAD: *The bread can be toasted up to a day in advance and kept in an airtight container at room temperature; the vegetables can be prepped up to a day in advance and stored in an airtight container in the fridge.*

FRIENDSGIVING PRO TIP

To make a vegan version, use browned cremini mushrooms instead of the sausage, vegetable stock, and a drizzle of oil at the end in place of the butter.

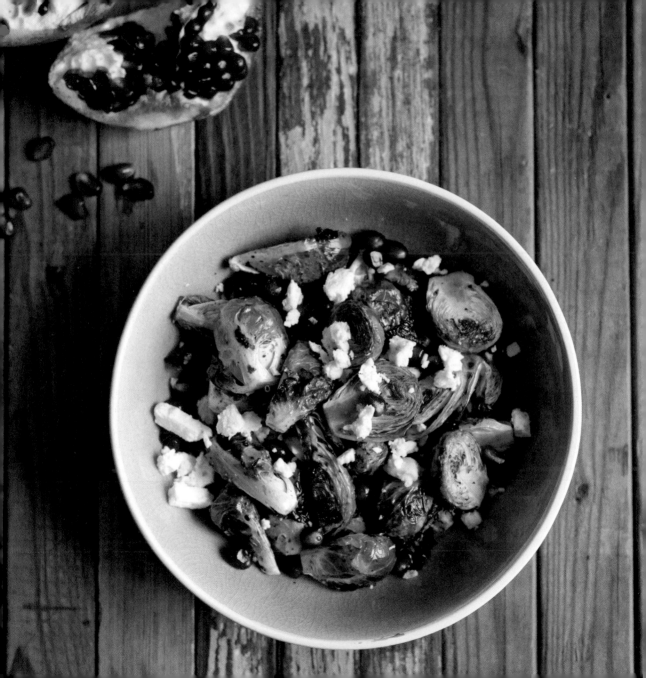

CHARRED BALSAMIC BRUSSELS SPROUTS WITH FETA AND POMEGRANATE SEEDS

MAKES 6 TO 8 SERVINGS

If overcooked or cooked incorrectly, Brussels sprouts can taste like gym socks. But if treated right, they can be as delicious and addictive as your favorite flavor of Doritos. The secret is cooking them on high heat—Brussels sprouts have got to be at least caramelized or, better still, charred. High heat also means less time on the stove or in the oven, so they retain most of their bite and don't turn into a mushy mess.

2 pounds Brussels sprouts, trimmed

¼ cup extra-virgin olive oil

½ teaspoon fine sea salt

¼ teaspoon freshly ground black pepper

2 tablespoons balsamic vinegar

4 ounces feta cheese, crumbled

¼ cup pomegranate seeds

1. Preheat the oven to 425°F.

2. Halve the smaller Brussels sprouts lengthwise and quarter the bigger ones. Toss with the oil, salt, and pepper to coat evenly. Divide between 2 baking sheets, spreading the Brussels sprouts into an even layer. Roast until crispy and dark brown, 15 to 20 minutes, tossing once halfway through cooking.

3. Transfer the Brussels sprouts to a large serving bowl and lightly toss with the balsamic vinegar. Top with the feta and pomegranate seeds. Serve immediately.

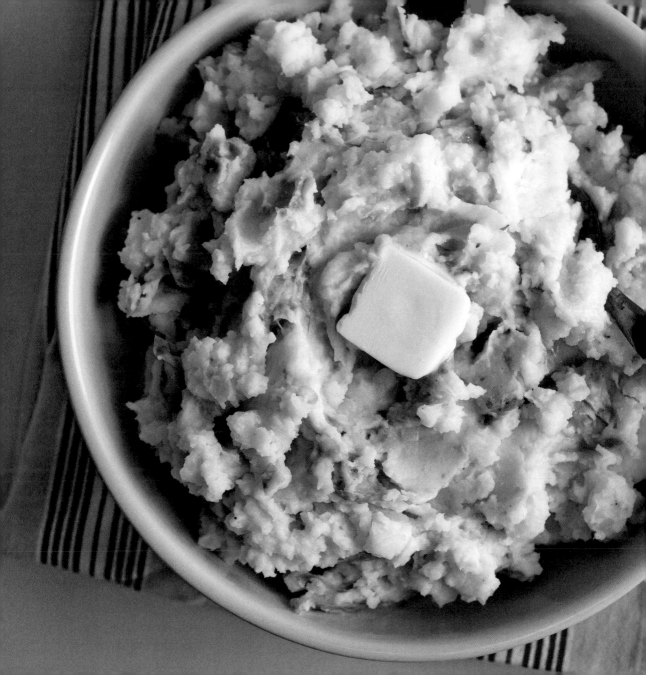

SOUR CREAM SMASHED POTATOES WITH FRIED SHALLOTS

MAKES 6 TO 8 SERVINGS

Regular mashed potatoes are great, but smashed potatoes cooked with their skins on are even better! They give the puree a chunkier texture with grooves that help catch the gravy you'll be pouring on. See? I've thought of everything.

3 pounds fingerling or other small potatoes, scrubbed and cut into 1-inch chunks

Sea salt

2 tablespoons canola oil

2 medium shallots, cut into half-moons

¾ cup whole milk

2 tablespoons (¼ stick) unsalted butter

¼ cup full-fat sour cream

Freshly ground black pepper

1. Place the potatoes into a large pot and add enough cold water to cover by about 2 inches. Add 2 teaspoons salt, cover tightly with a lid, and bring to a boil. Reduce the heat to low and simmer with the lid ajar until the potatoes can be easily pierced with a fork, about 20 minutes.

2. Meanwhile, heat the oil in a medium skillet over medium heat. Add the shallots and fry until dark caramel brown, about 4 minutes; set aside.

3. Combine the milk and butter in a small saucepan and warm over low heat until the butter is melted; set aside.

4. Drain the potatoes and transfer back to the pot. Lightly mash using a potato masher to break them up. Add the milk-butter mixture and sour cream. Continue mashing until everything comes together but some lumps of potato remain.

5. Stir in the shallots with their oil and season to taste with salt and pepper. Serve immediately.

LEFTOVER STRATEGY

Make croquettes! In a large bowl, stir 2 cups of the cold leftover potatoes with 1 beaten egg, 1 tablespoon all-purpose flour, and 1 cup mix-ins of your choice (cooked veggies, herbs, cheese, shredded turkey/roast pork, etc.). Form the mixture into 2-inch round patties, dredge in plain bread crumbs, and pan-fry in a bit of olive oil until golden brown and crispy. Serve with mashed avocado or spicy mayo, and a crunchy side salad.

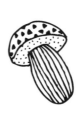
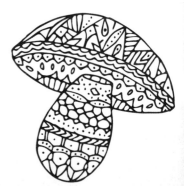

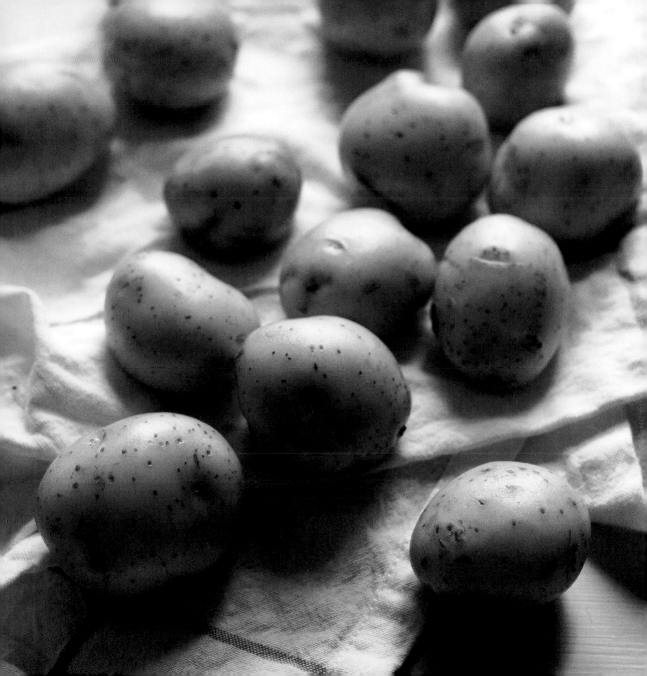

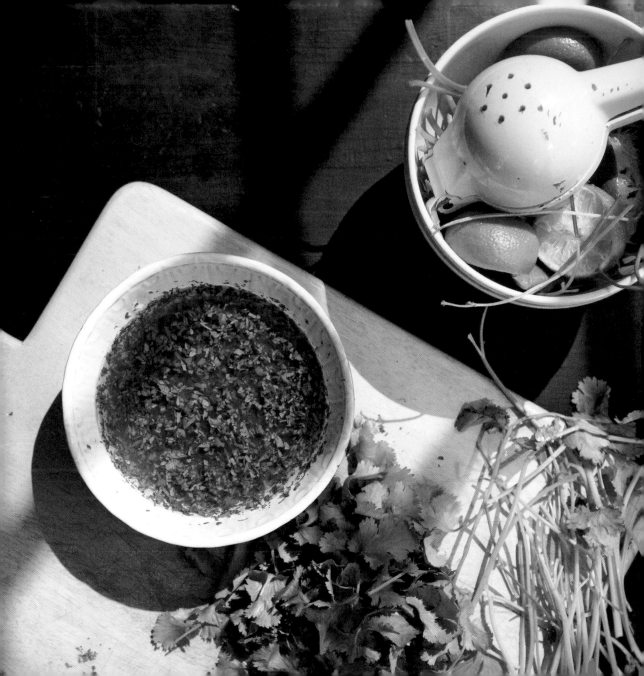

THE CUBAN FIESTA

The Cuban answer to meat and potatoes? Slow-roasted pork and creamy boiled yuca. This Cuban-inspired menu is an exciting departure from typical holiday food and a great way to introduce your friends to new flavors. Blast some Buena Vista Social Club, and keep the *mojitos* flowing!

Slow-Roasted Pork Shoulder
47

Yuca with Cilantro-Lime Mojo
50

Cuban-Style Refried Black Beans
49

Jicama, Avocado, and Mango Salad
52

TIMELINE

7 HOURS AHEAD: Start marinating the pork.

5 HOURS AHEAD: Start roasting the pork.

1.5 HOURS AHEAD: Make the refried beans.

1 HOUR AHEAD: Make the yuca, then the salad.

A LITTLE HELP FROM YOUR FRIENDS
Rum, limes, sugar, mint. Need I say more?

SUGGESTED WINE PAIRINGS
Pinot Noir or Tempranillo

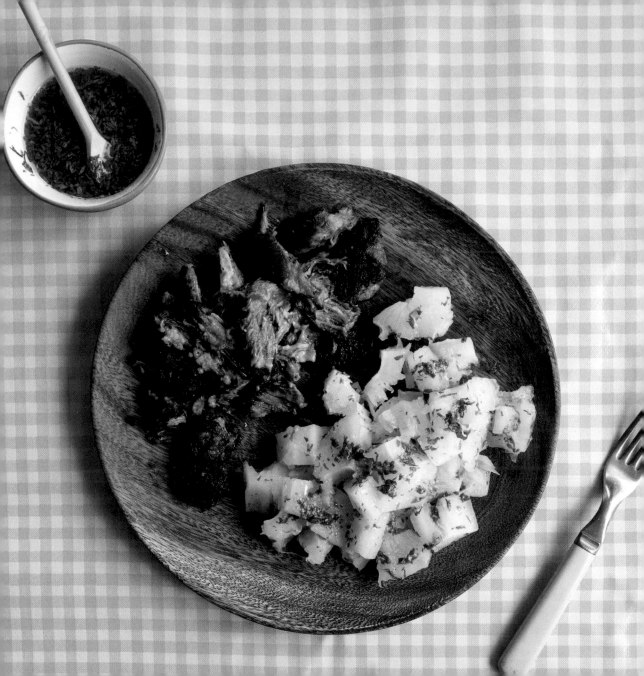

SLOW-ROASTED PORK SHOULDER

You'd think that something as delicious as this classic roasted pork requires a lot of time and energy to make, but you'd be wrong. The most difficult part of the whole ordeal is summoning enough patience to wait for it to finish cooking. Seriously, do not take the pork out of the oven until you are absolutely sure it is pull-apart, fork-tender.

5 large garlic cloves, minced

3 packed tablespoons minced fresh cilantro

2 tablespoons freshly squeezed lime juice (from 1 to 2 limes)

1 tablespoon white vinegar

1 tablespoon canola or other neutral oil

2 teaspoons ground cumin

1½ teaspoons fine sea salt

½ teaspoon coarsely ground black pepper

One 5- to 6-pound boneless pork shoulder

1. Whisk together the garlic, cilantro, lime juice, vinegar, oil, cumin, salt, and pepper in a small bowl; set aside.

2. Slice the pork skin diagonally at 1-inch intervals in both directions, creating a cross-hatch pattern. Place the pork into a Dutch oven or high-sided roasting pan skin side up and rub with the garlic marinade. Cover with a lid or foil, and chill for at least 2 hours or overnight.

3. Preheat the oven to 425°F.

4. Place the pork in the oven and reduce the heat to 300°F. Roast covered, basting the pork with its juices every hour or so, until the meat can be easily pierced with a knife with no resistance, 4 to 5 hours.

5. Uncover the pork and increase the temperature back to 425°F. Roast, basting every now and then, until the pork is brown and crisp, about 15 more minutes.

6. Remove the pork from the oven and let it rest uncovered for about 10 minutes. Shred it using a knife and fork.

 ## LEFTOVER STRATEGY

Cuban sandwiches! Pile leftover pork into Portuguese rolls slathered with yellow mustard, along with pickles, deli ham, and slices of mild, melty cheese. Cook in a lightly oiled skillet until hot and crisp.

CUBAN-STYLE REFRIED BLACK BEANS

This classic recipe is sure to become a staple in your meal-prep repertoire way beyond Friendsgiving. I love these in grain bowls, on sourdough toast, or topped with a fried egg for breakfast.

---

1 tablespoon canola oil

½ small onion, finely diced

Sea salt

3 medium garlic cloves, minced

1½ teaspoons ground cumin

Three 14-ounce cans no-salt-added black beans, drained and rinsed

¾ cup low-sodium vegetable stock

Freshly ground black pepper

2 teaspoons apple cider vinegar

1. Heat the oil in a medium saucepan over medium-low heat. Add the onion with a pinch of salt and cook until softened, about 4 minutes. Stir in the garlic and cumin, and cook for another minute.

2. Add half of the beans to the saucepan. Mash until most of the beans are crushed and pasty. Stir in the remaining beans and the vegetable stock. Season to taste with pinches of salt and pepper, cover tightly with a lid, and simmer for 10 minutes.

3. Stir in the vinegar. Season with more salt and pepper, if needed.

YUCA WITH CILANTRO-LIME MOJO

MAKES 6 TO 8 SERVINGS

Yuca (also known as cassava) is native to South America. It's a hard starchy vegetable with skin that looks like tree bark, so you wouldn't necessarily be drawn to it at the supermarket. When peeled and boiled, though, it most closely resembles a white potato but with an even waxier, creamier texture and sweeter flavor, which is why I find it totally irresistible. *See photo on page 46.*

4 medium yuca stalks (about 3 pounds; see Note)

Sea salt

½ recipe Cilantro-Lime Mojo (recipe follows)

1. Using a sharp knife, cut the yuca crosswise into 2 or 3 pieces so it is easier to manage. Stand each piece on a flat side and slice off the tough skin. Cut each piece lengthwise into quarters. The center of the yuca has a tough fibrous core—slice ¼ inch off from the center of each quarter and discard. Cut each resulting baton of yuca into ¾-inch pieces.

2. Place the yuca into a large pot. Add enough water to cover by 2 inches, along with a generous pinch of salt. Cover tightly with a lid and bring to a boil. Reduce the heat to low and simmer with the lid ajar until the yuca can be pierced with a fork, like soft butter, about 15 minutes.

3. Drain the yuca and return to the pot. Drizzle with *mojo* and toss to coat. Transfer to a serving dish and serve immediately.

NOTE: *If your yuca has brown spots or smells strongly acidic when you cut into it, it's no longer fresh. Can't find yuca at your local store? Use white potatoes instead.*

CILANTRO-LIME MOJO

Serve the leftover *mojo* with Slow-Roasted Pork Shoulder (page 47).

½ cup freshly squeezed lime juice (from 6 limes)

½ cup canola or other neutral oil

4 small garlic cloves, crushed or mashed into a paste

¼ cup packed minced fresh cilantro

1 teaspoon fine sea salt

Whisk together the lime juice, oil, garlic, cilantro, and salt in a small bowl.

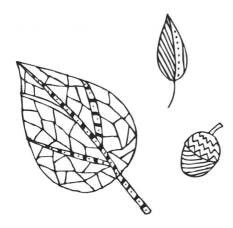

JICAMA, AVOCADO, AND MANGO SALAD

Jicama is a vegetable native to Mexico. It's crunchy, juicy, and best eaten raw, which makes it a refreshing, palate-cleansing addition to this meal. Paired with creamy avocado and sweet mango, the salad adds lightness to this otherwise heavy menu.

---

3 tablespoons freshly squeezed lime juice (from about 2 limes)

2 tablespoons canola oil

2 packed tablespoons minced fresh cilantro

½ small garlic clove, minced

½ teaspoon fine sea salt

1 large jicama bulb (about 2 pounds), peeled and cut into ⅓-inch cubes

2 small ripe avocados, pitted, peeled, and cut into ⅓-inch cubes

2 small ripe mangoes, pitted, peeled, and cut into ⅓-inch cubes

1. Whisk together the lime juice, oil, cilantro, garlic, and salt in a small bowl.

2. Place the cubed jicama, avocados, and mangoes into a large bowl. Toss with the dressing to combine and serve immediately.

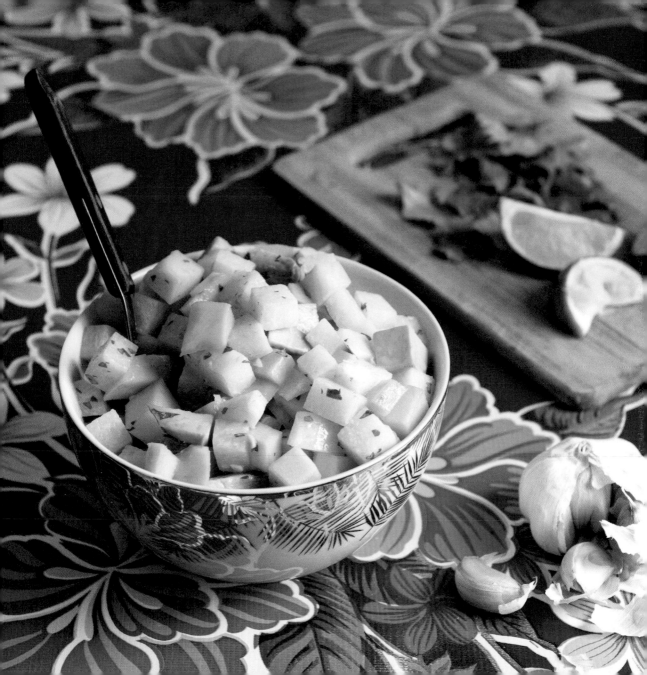

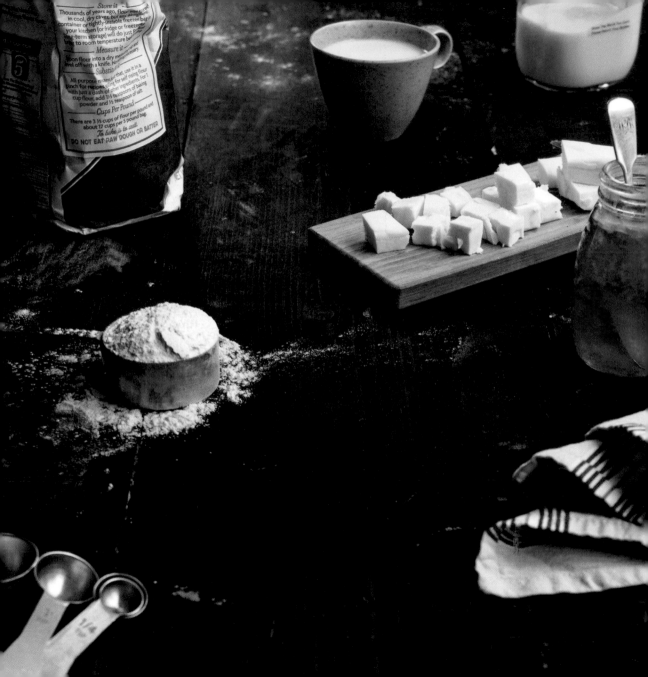

THE SOUTHERN FEAST

Crunchy fried chicken, buttery biscuits, irresistibly savory tomato pudding
(wait till you taste this thing!), and a tangy slaw. This stick-to-your bones menu is
so satisfying, you may not go back to turkey for years to come . . . or like, ever.

**Buttermilk Fried Chicken
with Spicy Honey**
57

**Purple Cabbage Slaw with
Lemon-Dill Yogurt Dressing**
59

Southern Tomato Pudding
60

**Buttermilk Biscuits with Lemon Zest–
Black Pepper Compound Butter**
63

TIMELINE

3 HOURS AHEAD: Start marinating the chicken and make the spicy honey and compound butter.

2 HOURS AHEAD: Make the tomato pudding.

1 HOUR AHEAD: Shred the cabbage, make the yogurt dressing, and start frying the chicken.

RIGHT BEFORE GUESTS ARRIVE: Make the biscuits and toss the salad.

A LITTLE HELP FROM YOUR FRIENDS

Pimento cheese is a perfect complement to this meal. Ask a friend to make it from scratch!

SUGGESTED WINE PAIRINGS

Riesling or a dry rosé

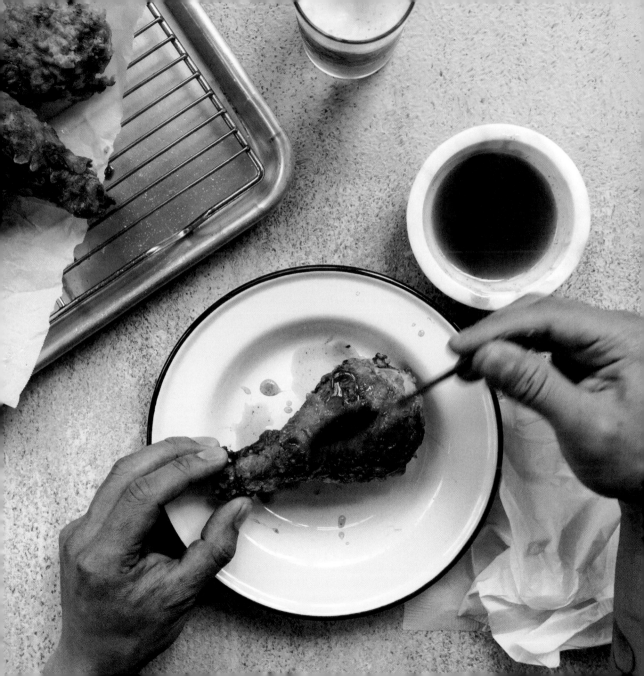

BUTTERMILK FRIED CHICKEN WITH SPICY HONEY

Under no circumstances should you let guests into the kitchen while you fry, or there will be no chicken left to bring to the table. You've been warned.

CHICKEN

3 pounds skin-on, bone-in chicken drumsticks and thighs (16 pieces in total), patted dry

About 6 cups buttermilk

2½ cups all-purpose flour

3 teaspoons garlic powder

2½ teaspoons sea salt

2½ teaspoons coarsely ground black pepper

1½ teaspoons smoked paprika

About 4 cups peanut oil, for frying

1. Place the chicken in a large shallow container and pour in the buttermilk, making sure all the pieces are submerged. Cover the container tightly with plastic wrap and refrigerate for 1 hour.

2. In the meantime, make the spicy honey: Whisk together the honey, hot sauce, salt, and pepper in a small bowl. Taste and adjust seasonings, if needed. Transfer to a small serving bowl, cover, and set aside until ready to serve.

3. Remove the chicken from the fridge and let it stand at room temperature while you get ready to fry. Fit a cooling rack within a large baking sheet and set aside.

4. Whisk together the flour, garlic powder, salt, pepper, and paprika in a separate shallow dish.

5. Heat the oil in a large cast-iron skillet or another high-sided, heavy-bottomed pan over medium heat, making sure there is enough oil to come at least halfway up the chicken once you add it in, about 1½ inches. When the oil

continues on next page

SPICY HONEY

1 cup honey

4 teaspoons Louisiana-style hot sauce or to taste

Pinches of sea salt and freshly ground black pepper

is hot, working with 1 piece at a time, lift the chicken out of the buttermilk and shake off the excess. Dredge the chicken in the flour mixture, making sure to firmly press the flour into the chicken to form a generous coating.

6. Carefully place the chicken in the hot oil. Repeat with the remaining chicken, frying about 4 pieces at a time, making sure not to overcrowd the pan. Fry for 8 to 10 minutes, until the chicken turns a deep golden brown color underneath. (If the chicken is browning too quickly, reduce the heat a bit. If the chicken is not yet ready, resist the urge to flip.) Using tongs, carefully turn the chicken, and cook the other side for another 8 to 10 minutes; again, resist the urge to flip.

7. Transfer to the prepared cooling rack and repeat with the remaining chicken. Transfer to a serving dish and serve immediately with the spicy honey dip.

DO AHEAD: *The spicy honey can be made up to several days in advance and stored in an airtight container at room temperature.*

FRIENDSGIVING PRO TIP

The chicken is, of course, best eaten immediately. In case dinner gets delayed, keep the chicken warm in a 150° to 200°F oven.

PURPLE CABBAGE SLAW
WITH LEMON-DILL YOGURT DRESSING

MAKES 6 TO 8 SERVINGS

This cooling yogurt dressing and the crunchy veggies are a nice way to offset the weightiness of the other recipes in this menu. For uniformly shredded cabbage and to save time, shred it in the food processor using the shredding attachment.

---

1 cup plain full-fat Greek yogurt

3 tablespoons freshly squeezed lemon juice (from about 1½ lemons)

3 packed tablespoons chopped fresh dill

Fine sea salt

2 medium carrots, cut into short matchsticks

1 medium purple cabbage (about 2 pounds), cored and finely shredded

1. Stir together the yogurt, lemon juice, dill, and ½ teaspoon of the salt in a large bowl.

2. Toss the carrots and cabbage with the dressing right before serving. Taste and adjust seasoning, if needed.

SOUTHERN TOMATO PUDDING

My boyfriend and I love to go on road trips, and scenic Charleston, South Carolina, is one of our favorite stops. The place where we typically stay is right around the corner from the famed Hominy Grill, a cozy restaurant that serves southern classics, like fried chicken, biscuits, collard greens, and the lesser known tomato pudding. It's a very simple dish of bread, tomato sauce, butter, and sugar, baked to sweet, saucy perfection. I know it sounds a little weird, but trust me, there is no better accompaniment to salty chicken than sweet tomato pudding.

---

4 slices white sandwich bread, torn into ½-inch pieces (see Note)

3 tablespoons unsalted butter, melted

One 28-ounce can tomato puree

¼ cup sugar

¼ teaspoon fine sea salt

1. Preheat the oven to 375°F.

2. Place the bread in an 8 × 8-inch baking dish and drizzle with butter. Toss to coat and set aside.

3. Stir together the tomato puree, sugar, and salt in a large bowl.

4. Pour the tomato mixture over the bread and shake the dish to help the tomatoes settle. Bake until bubbly and golden brown, 30 to 35 minutes.

NOTE: *Use the plainest white sandwich bread you can find—meaning the stuff from the supermarket aisle, not the bakery section.*

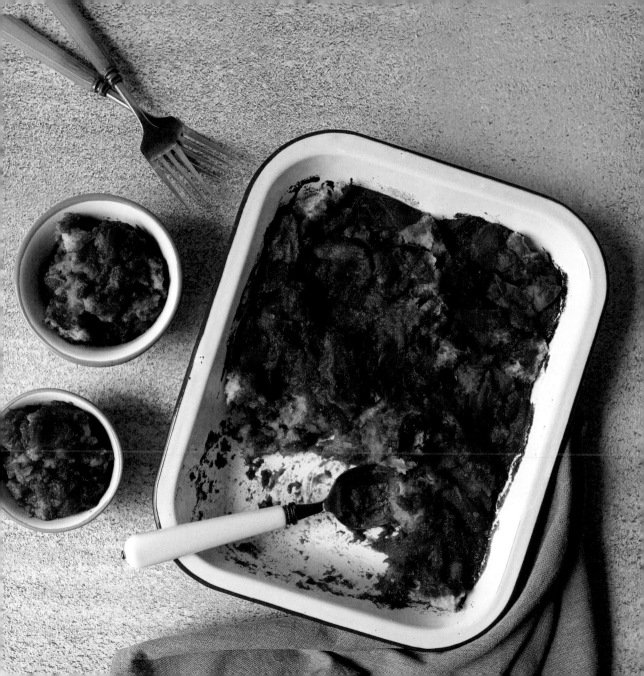

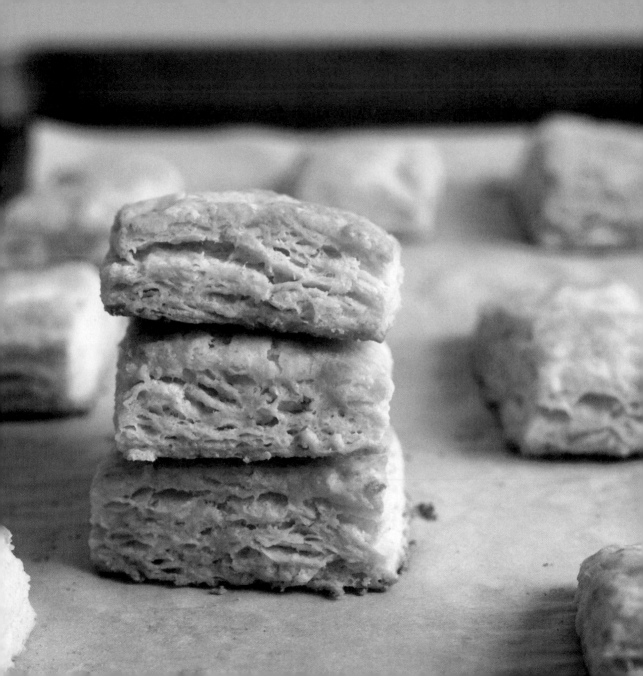

BUTTERMILK BISCUITS WITH LEMON ZEST–BLACK PEPPER COMPOUND BUTTER

MAKES 16 BISCUITS

The objective with biscuit dough is to have really flaky biscuits. This is done by using really cold butter and really cold buttermilk, and being careful not to work the dough too much. These biscuits are best served straight out of the oven, so I recommend baking them after your guests have already arrived.

BISCUITS

2 cups all-purpose flour, plus more for dusting

1 tablespoon baking powder

½ teaspoon baking soda

½ teaspoon fine sea salt

1 stick (4 ounces) cold unsalted butter (see Note, page 64)

1 cup cold buttermilk

COMPOUND BUTTER

6 tablespoons (¾ stick) unsalted butter, at room temperature

Zest of 1 lemon (about 1½ teaspoons)

continues on next page

1. Preheat the oven to 425°F. Line a baking sheet with parchment paper and set aside.

2. Combine the flour, baking powder, baking soda, and salt in a large bowl and whisk to combine.

3. Using the large-hole side of a box grater, grate the butter into the flour mixture. Toss the mixture with your hands to evenly distribute the butter and coat it in flour. Refrigerate for 5 minutes.

4. Add the buttermilk to the flour-butter mixture and toss with a rubber spatula until a shaggy dough forms. Turn the dough out onto a lightly floured surface, gently knead it a few times until it comes together, and roll it out into a 1-inch-thick rectangle.

   Fold the dough in half so that the short ends meet and roll it out again. Fold it one more time and roll the dough out into an 8-inch square (about 1 inch thick). Cut the dough into 16 square biscuits.

½ teaspoon freshly ground
black pepper

¼ teaspoon fine sea salt

5. Transfer the biscuit squares to the prepared baking sheet and bake until the biscuits are golden brown, 12 to 15 minutes.

6. Make the compound butter: In a small bowl, mash the butter, lemon zest, pepper, and salt with a fork until evenly combined. Place the bowl in the freezer for a few minutes to solidify the butter a bit. Scrape the butter onto the center of a sheet of parchment paper and gently form into a log with your hands. Fold the long edges of the parchment paper to meet on top and roll the butter into a circular log inside the paper. Refrigerate until solidified, about 10 minutes. Slice into thin rounds before serving.

7. Serve the hot biscuits immediately alongside the compound butter.

NOTE: *To get the butter appropriately cold for grating, I place it in the freezer for 5 to 10 minutes.*

DO AHEAD: *The compound butter can be made up to several days in advance.*

 FRIENDSGIVING PRO TIP

For other variations of compound butter, try swapping out the lemon zest and black pepper for a sweeter version with dashes of cinnamon and maple syrup or an herby blend of chopped fresh dill and chives.

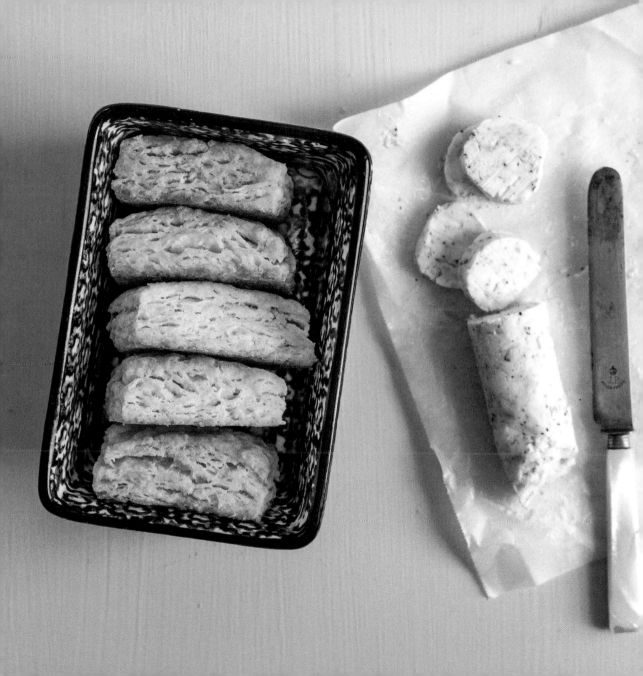

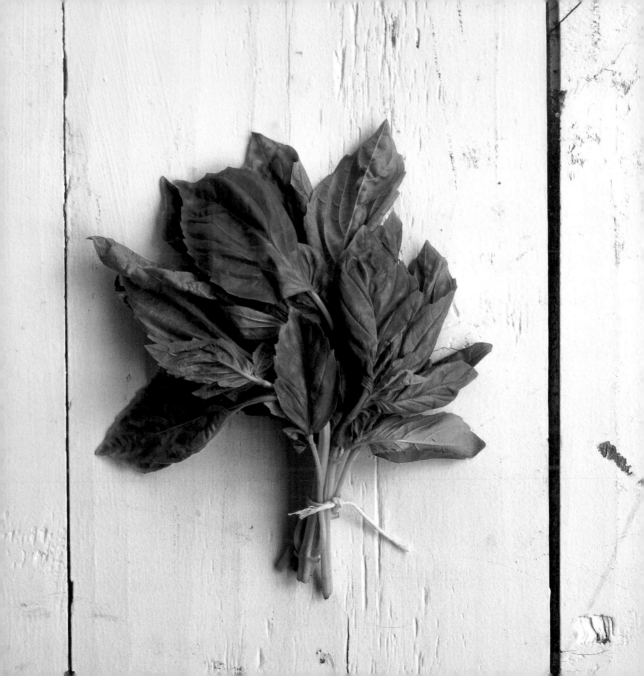

THE NONNA SPECIAL

Fact: Everyone loves Italian-American food. If you've got picky eaters—
or friends with kids!—at the table, this menu is the way to go. You just can't go
wrong by bringing the red-sauce joint home.

**Stewed White Beans
with Garlic and Rosemary**
68

**Kale and Butternut Squash Salad with
Spicy Seeds and Goat Cheese**
71

**Chicken Parmesan with
Homemade Bread Crumbs and
Red Sauce**
73

Spaghetti Pie
77

TIMELINE

1 DAY AHEAD: Soak the beans.

2 HOURS AHEAD: Roast the squash, and start cooking the beans.

1.5 HOURS AHEAD: Make the chicken Parmesan.

1 HOUR AHEAD: Make the spaghetti pie, then finish the salad.

A LITTLE HELP FROM YOUR FRIENDS

Ask for fancy bottles of olive oil and balsamic vinegar and a few loaves of
focaccia for dipping.

SUGGESTED WINE PAIRINGS

Chardonnay or Chianti

STEWED WHITE BEANS WITH GARLIC AND ROSEMARY

Much like the Cuban-Style Refried Black Beans (page 49), these beans are likely to become a staple in your kitchen. I love to make a big pot of them on Sunday and eat them throughout the week on toast, in salads, or in grain bowls.

3 tablespoons extra-virgin olive oil

1 head of garlic, papery outermost layer peeled away, then halved widthwise

¼ teaspoon red pepper flakes

1½ cups dried cannellini beans, soaked for at least 8 hours or overnight, drained, and rinsed

1 fresh rosemary sprig

One 2-inch piece of Parmesan rind (optional)

Sea salt and coarsely ground black pepper

1. Heat 1 tablespoon of the oil in a Dutch oven or large pot over medium-low heat. Add the garlic halves cut side down and cook until they are nicely browned, 2 to 3 minutes, being careful not to burn. Add the red pepper flakes and cook for another 30 seconds.

2. Add the beans, rosemary, Parmesan rind (if using), 1 tablespoon salt, a few grinds of black pepper, and enough water to cover by about 2 inches. Cover tightly with a lid and bring to a boil. Reduce the heat to low and simmer until the beans are soft and creamy, 45 to 60 minutes.

3. Pour out most of the cooking water and discard, leaving only enough to keep the beans saucy but not soupy. Pull out the garlic, rosemary, and Parmesan rind and discard. Stir in the remaining 2 tablespoons oil and season to taste with salt and pepper.

LEFTOVER STRATEGY

Top warmed beans with a crispy fried egg and a handful of arugula, and serve with pan-toasted ciabatta bread for a hearty breakfast or brunch.

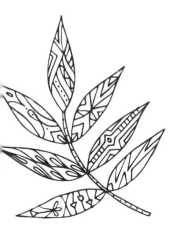

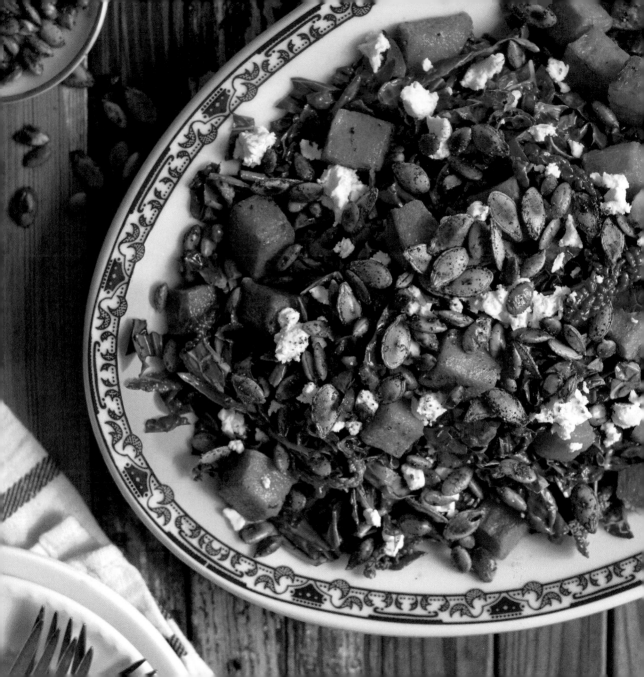

KALE AND BUTTERNUT SQUASH SALAD WITH SPICY SEEDS AND GOAT CHEESE

Dissecting and cooking a whole butternut squash may seem a little scary because of its large size and irregular shape. One way to set yourself up for success is to use a sharp chef's knife. Once the squash is cubed, the rest is a breeze. Make extra spiced seeds to use as part of the Choose-Your-Own-Adventure Crostini Bar (page 19) or the Cheese Board (page 103).

---

1 medium butternut squash (about 2½ pounds)

¼ cup extra-virgin olive oil

Sea salt and freshly ground black pepper

2 tablespoons shelled pumpkin seeds

½ teaspoon unrefined coconut oil or extra-virgin olive oil

¼ teaspoon smoked paprika

¼ teaspoon garlic powder

2 bunches of lacinato kale, stemmed and sliced into thin ribbons

continues on next page

1. Preheat the oven to 400°F. Line a baking sheet with parchment paper and set aside.

2. Using a sharp knife, trim the top and bottom of the squash, then halve it widthwise, separating the thinner top from the bigger bottom half. Stand halves on a flat side and slice off the skin, running your knife from top to bottom around the squash. Discard the skin. Halve the bottom portion lengthwise, and using a tablespoon, scrape out and reserve the seeds. Cut all the squash into 1-inch cubes and place into a large bowl. Drizzle with 2 tablespoons of the olive oil, ¼ teaspoon salt, and a few grinds of pepper and toss to coat. Transfer to the prepared baking sheet and spread into an even layer. Roast for 25 to 30 minutes, tossing once halfway through cooking, until the squash is tender and lightly browned.

3 tablespoons balsamic
vinegar

2 ounces goat cheese,
crumbled

3. Meanwhile, pick out the reserved squash seeds (you should have about 2 tablespoons of seeds), discarding any squash strings. Place the seeds in a colander and rinse under running water. Transfer the seeds to a kitchen towel and pat dry. Place the seeds in a small skillet and toast over low heat until they are slightly puffy and smell nutty, about 5 minutes. Add the shelled pumpkin seeds and continue toasting for another few minutes. Add the coconut oil and toss to coat. Season with the paprika, garlic, and ¼ teaspoon salt. Transfer to a bowl and set aside.

4. Place the kale in a large mixing bowl and drizzle with the balsamic vinegar, the remaining 2 tablespoons of olive oil, and a generous pinch of salt. Using your hands, massage the kale until it is softened and darkened in color, 1 to 2 minutes.

5. Transfer the kale to a serving platter and top with the roasted squash, spiced seeds, and goat cheese. Serve immediately.

DO AHEAD: *The butternut squash can be cooked up to a day in advance and stored in an airtight container in the fridge. Reheat slightly before adding to the salad.*

CHICKEN PARMESAN
WITH HOMEMADE BREAD CRUMBS AND RED SAUCE

MAKES 8 SERVINGS

The key to good chicken Parm is practicing restraint with sauce and cheese. You do not want the chicken disintegrating in a sea of red—just a light coating will do. A few extra steps can also help take things to the next level—like using fresh bread crumbs, which creates a nice thick coating, and grating your own cheese instead of using pregrated, which is typically processed with extra additives. To make the cheese easier to grate, place it in the freezer for a couple of minutes.

RED SAUCE

1 tablespoon extra-virgin olive oil

2 large garlic cloves, minced

Pinch of red pepper flakes

One 28-ounce can no-salt-added crushed tomatoes

¾ teaspoon sugar

Sea salt and freshly ground black pepper

About 8 basil leaves, torn

continues on next page

1. Make the red sauce: Heat the oil in a medium pot over low heat. Add the garlic and red pepper flakes and cook for about 1 minute. Add the tomatoes, sugar, ¼ teaspoon salt, and a few grinds of pepper. Cover, bring to a simmer, and cook for 10 minutes, stirring occasionally. Turn the heat off and stir in the basil. Taste and adjust seasonings, if needed.

2. Ladle a bit of the tomato sauce into a baking dish and spread to cover the bottom. Reserve the remaining sauce.

3. Make the bread crumbs: Place the bread in a food processor and pulverize into a fine meal—you should have about 3 cups of bread crumbs. Transfer to a shallow dish, mix in the thyme and rosemary, and set aside.

About 6 slices of day-old
white bread

2 fresh thyme sprigs, leaves
picked and minced (about
1 teaspoon)

1 fresh rosemary sprig,
leaves picked and minced
(about 1½ teaspoons)

About ¼ cup extra-virgin
olive oil

4 skinless, boneless chicken
breasts (about 2 pounds),
halved widthwise to form
8 cutlets

Sea salt and freshly ground
black pepper

3 ounces mozzarella cheese,
grated (about 1 cup)

2 ounces Parmesan cheese,
grated (about ¾ cup)

4. Preheat the oven to 375°F.

5. Heat about 2 tablespoons of the oil in a large nonstick
skillet over medium-high heat. Season the chicken with
salt and pepper on both sides, and dredge it in the bread
crumb mixture. Fry 2 to 3 cutlets at a time (making sure
not to overcrowd the skillet) until golden brown, about
2 minutes. Flip using tongs and brown the other side.
Transfer browned cutlets to the prepared baking dish
and continue cooking the rest of the chicken, adding
more oil to the skillet as needed.

6. Ladle a bit of the sauce on the chicken and top with
the mozzarella and Parmesan. Bake until the cheese is
melted and starting to brown, 20 to 25 minutes. Serve
immediately.

NOTE: *This tomato sauce recipe makes enough for both the
chicken and the Spaghetti Pie (page 77).*

DO AHEAD: *The sauce will keep in an airtight container in
the fridge for up to 4 days.*

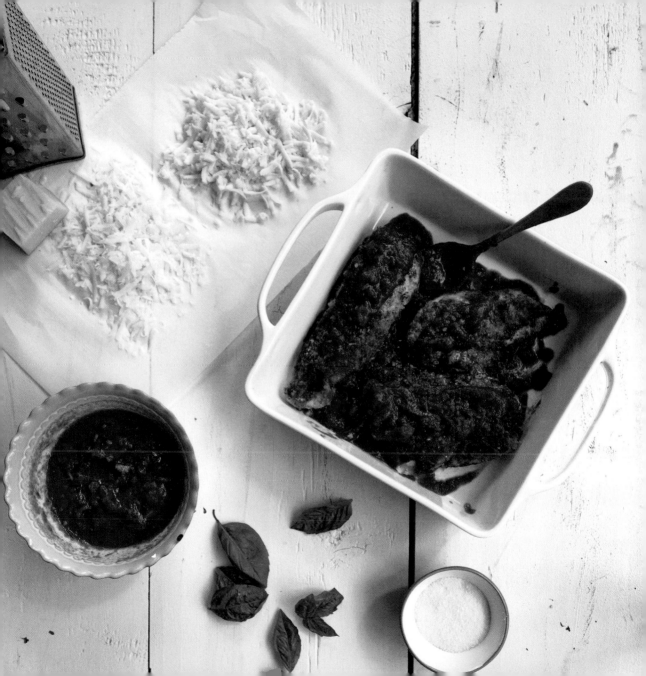

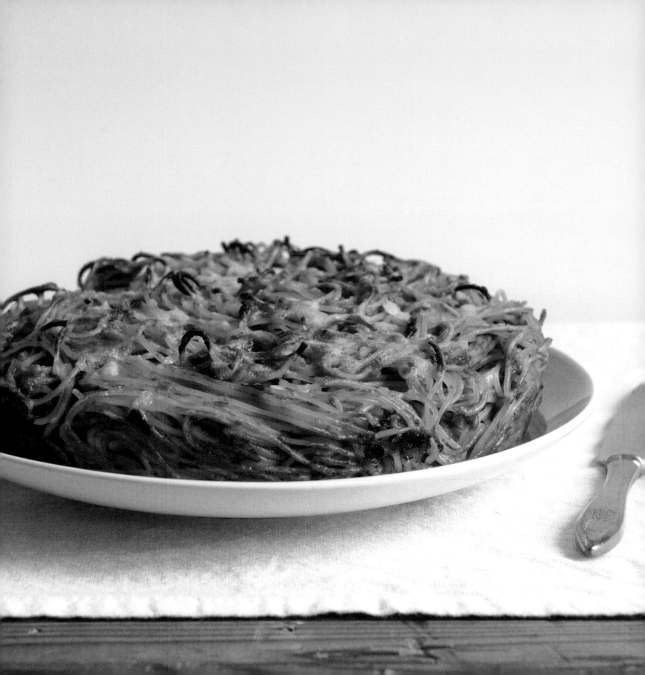

SPAGHETTI PIE

Meet your new favorite pasta dish. It's spaghetti, in the shape of a pie, with crispy edges and a chewy interior. This dish is as fun as it is tasty—your friends could eat it with their hands if they wanted to.

---

1 pound good-quality spaghetti

1 tablespoon butter

3 large eggs, beaten

1 cup homemade red sauce (see page 73) or prepared tomato sauce

¼ teaspoon coarsely ground black pepper

Pinch of salt

3 ounces mozzarella cheese, grated (about 1 cup)

1½ ounces Parmesan cheese, grated (about ½ cup)

1. Cook the pasta in generously salted water according to the package directions until just shy of al dente. Drain and set aside.

2. Preheat the oven to 400°F. Butter a 9-inch springform pan (see Note) and set aside.

3. In a large bowl, stir together the eggs, red sauce, pepper, salt, and all but 1 tablespoon each of the mozzarella and Parmesan. Add the pasta and toss to coat evenly. Transfer to the prepared springform pan and sprinkle with the reserved cheeses.

4. Bake until the top is nicely browned and crisp, 30 to 35 minutes. Let cool for 5 minutes before unmolding.

NOTE: *If you don't own a springform pan, feel free to use any round baking dish and serve the pie directly out of it.*

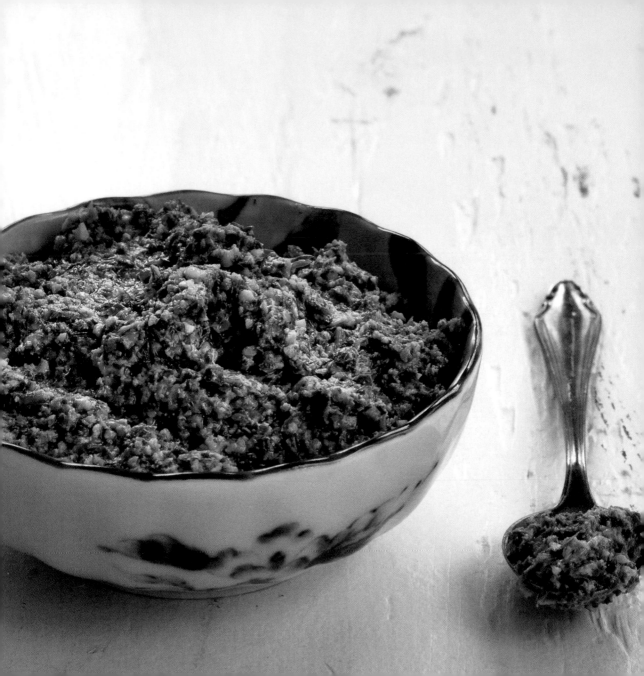

THE MODERN

Whether you and your friends are typical health nuts or not, a holiday party is a great time to experiment with new techniques and healthier recipes. This vegan, gluten-free menu is sure to please everyone at your table.

Garlicky Chickpea-Celeriac Puree 80	**Roasted Cauliflower Steaks with Arugula-Walnut Pesto** 85
Crunchy Stuffed Cremini Mushrooms 82	**Frisée Salad with Warm Shiitake Dressing and Pine Nuts** 87

TIMELINE

1 DAY AHEAD: Soak the chickpeas and cashews for the puree.

2 HOURS AHEAD: Start making the puree, then the stuffed mushrooms and the pesto.

1 HOUR AHEAD. Roast the cauliflower, then make the salad.

A LITTLE HELP FROM YOUR FRIENDS

Hummus, baba ghanoush, and freshly baked gluten-free bread from your favorite bakery would be welcome contributions.

SUGGESTED WINE PAIRINGS

Sauvignon Blanc or Pinot Noir

GARLICKY CHICKPEA-CELERIAC PUREE

Celeriac (also known as celery root) is the bottom portion of the green celery we're all familiar with. It's a round vegetable with irregularly shaped grooves on the skin that are best peeled with a sharp chef's knife. It's creamy and sweet with a very mild celery flavor that's more interesting for a festive get-together than regular ol' potatoes.

I know you're probably wondering if you can use canned chickpeas. The answer is yeah, sure, but I find that canned chickpeas always taste like the can and not like the creamy nutty things they're supposed to be. With that said, in a pinch, you can warm 3 cups of well-rinsed and drained canned chickpeas before adding them to the puree.

---

1 cup dried chickpeas, soaked for at least 8 hours or overnight, drained, and rinsed

2 medium garlic cloves, smashed and halved

Sea salt

2 large celeriac bulbs (2½ pounds), peeled and cut into 1-inch chunks

½ cup raw cashews, soaked for at least 4 hours or overnight and drained

2 tablespoons extra-virgin olive oil

1. Place the chickpeas and garlic in a medium pot, along with a teaspoon of salt and enough cold water to cover by about 2 inches. Cover and bring to a boil, then reduce the heat to low and simmer with the lid ajar until the chickpeas have a creamy texture, about 40 minutes.

2. Meanwhile, place the celeriac in a separate medium pot. Add a teaspoon of salt and enough cold water to cover by about 2 inches. Cover and bring to a boil, then reduce the heat to low and simmer with the lid ajar until the celeriac can be pierced very easily with a fork, about 20 minutes. Reserve about ½ cup of the cooking water and drain the celeriac.

3. Drain the chickpeas, then puree the ingredients in 2 batches. Start by combining half of the chickpeas

4 teaspoons white miso

Freshly ground black pepper

with half of the celeriac and half of the cashews in a food processor and puree. Add a tablespoon of oil, 2 teaspoons of the miso, and 1 tablespoon of the reserved celeriac cooking water and puree until completely smooth, 1 to 2 minutes, adding more celeriac cooking water if needed to achieve the desired consistency. Season with salt and pepper to taste and puree for another few seconds. Transfer to a bowl and repeat with the other half of the ingredients. Combine the purees. Serve immediately.

DO AHEAD: *The chickpeas can be cooked a day in advance, allowed to cool, then stored with their cooking liquid in an airtight container in the fridge. Reheat before pureeing.*

 ## LEFTOVER STRATEGY

The puree keeps pretty well in the fridge for up to 4 days. Serve leftovers with tomato-stewed lentils or roasted vegetables.

CRUNCHY STUFFED CREMINI MUSHROOMS

Bite-size and crispy, these mushrooms are always a crowd favorite. The star ingredient here is the nutritional yeast, a plant-based ingredient that has the power to add a savory, cheesy flavor to basically anything.

1½ pounds small fresh cremini mushrooms

¾ cup gluten-free panko bread crumbs

¼ cup nutritional yeast flakes

3 packed tablespoons minced fresh flat-leaf parsley

1 large garlic clove, minced

Zest of ½ lemon

½ teaspoon fine sea salt

¼ teaspoon freshly ground black pepper

⅓ cup extra-virgin olive oil

1. Preheat the oven to 350°F. Line a baking sheet with parchment paper and set aside.

2. Pop out the stems of the mushrooms and discard. Wipe the mushroom caps clean with a damp paper towel and place round side down on the prepared baking sheet and set aside.

3. Combine the bread crumbs, nutritional yeast, parsley, garlic, lemon zest, salt, pepper, and 2 tablespoons of the oil in a bowl.

4. Using a teaspoon measure, stuff each mushroom cap with a heaping mound of the bread crumb filling. Lightly drizzle the mushrooms with the remaining oil. Bake until golden brown, 20 to 25 minutes. Transfer to a serving platter and serve immediately.

DO AHEAD: *The mushrooms can be cleaned and stemmed, and the bread crumb filling made, up to a day in advance and stored in airtight containers in the fridge. That way all you have to do before the party is stuff and bake them!*

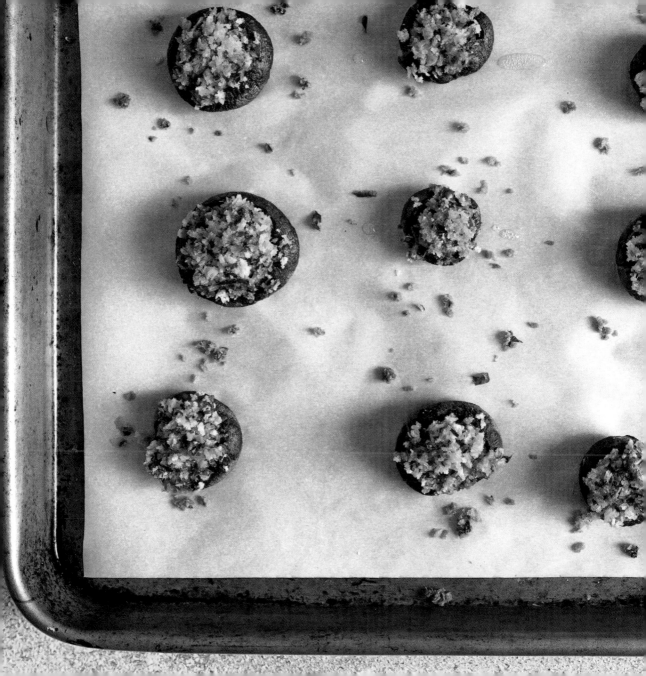

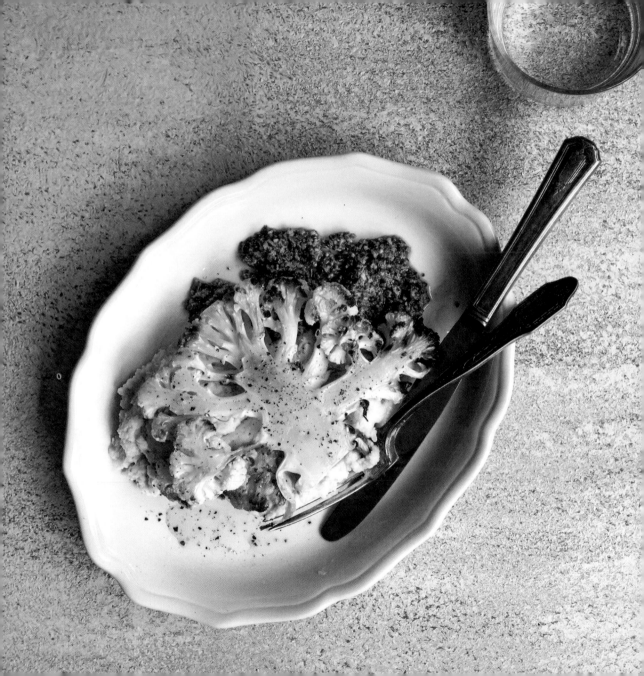

ROASTED CAULIFLOWER STEAKS WITH ARUGULA-WALNUT PESTO

MAKES 8 SERVINGS

This show-stopping main is a veggie-friendly alternative to turkey. Cauliflower is cheap, versatile, and takes on the flavor of anything it's paired with. Not a fan of pesto? These "steaks" also go well with Muhammara (page 24).

CAULIFLOWER

3 large heads of cauliflower

About 3 tablespoons extra-virgin olive oil

Sea salt and freshly ground black pepper

ARUGULA-WALNUT PESTO

3 cups packed arugula

½ cup packed fresh basil leaves

½ cup walnuts, toasted

1 tablespoon drained capers

1½ teaspoons white miso

1 medium garlic clove, roughly chopped

continues on next page

1. Preheat the oven to 425°F. Line 2 baking sheets with parchment paper and set aside.

2. Trim the bottom stem of the cauliflower, stand it on its flat bottom, and slice it into three ½-inch-thick planks (reserve the florets that become detached). Repeat with the remaining cauliflower. Lightly coat the planks with oil and season both sides with salt and pepper. Lay the cauliflower planks in a single layer on the prepared baking sheets. Toss the reserved florets with a bit of oil, salt, and pepper, and scatter them around the baking sheets.

3. Roast for 10 minutes, flip, and continue roasting until the steaks are browned around the edges, about 10 more minutes.

4. Meanwhile, make the pesto: Combine the arugula, basil, walnuts, capers, miso, garlic, and a few pinches of salt and pepper in a food processor. Pulse until everything

Sea salt and freshly ground
pepper

1 tablespoon freshly
squeezed lemon juice

⅓ cup extra-virgin olive oil

is broken down. With the motor running, stream in the lemon juice, then the oil, and puree until smooth. Season to taste with more salt and pepper, if needed. Scrape into a serving bowl and refrigerate until ready to serve.

5. Serve cauliflower steaks hot, alongside the arugula-walnut pesto with Garlicky Celeriac-Chickpea Puree (page 80), if desired.

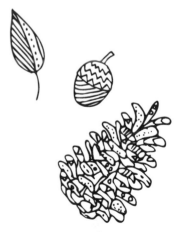

FRISÉE SALAD
WITH WARM SHIITAKE DRESSING AND PINE NUTS

MAKES 6 TO 8 SERVINGS

This salad is inspired by one of my favorite French dishes, *salade lyonnaise*, which consists of bitter frisée tossed in a warm bacon–Dijon mustard dressing and topped with a poached egg. This vegan version uses finely diced shiitake mushrooms to make an equally savory dressing. It's the perfect way to add a little—for lack of a better term—meatiness to this vegan menu.

¼ cup pine nuts

¾ pound fresh shiitake mushrooms, stemmed

¼ cup extra-virgin olive oil

2 small shallots, finely diced

3 tablespoons white wine or red wine vinegar

2 tablespoons Dijon mustard

Fine sea salt and freshly ground black pepper

2 heads of frisée (about 1½ pounds), torn into bite-size pieces (see Note)

1. Place the pine nuts in a small skillet and toast over medium-low heat until lightly golden, tossing occasionally, about 4 minutes. Set aside.

2. Wipe the mushroom caps clean with a damp paper towel and dice them finely.

3. Heat 2 tablespoons of the oil in a large nonstick skillet and add the mushrooms. Cook, stirring occasionally, until the mushrooms are nicely browned, 8 to 10 minutes. Add the shallots and cook for another minute. Remove from the heat and stir in the vinegar, mustard, and the remaining 2 tablespoons oil. Season to taste with salt and pepper.

4. Place the frisée in a large bowl and pour in the warm dressing. Toss to combine and top with the pine nuts. Serve immediately.

NOTE: *If you can't find frisée, use a mixture of finely shredded romaine and radicchio or endive.*

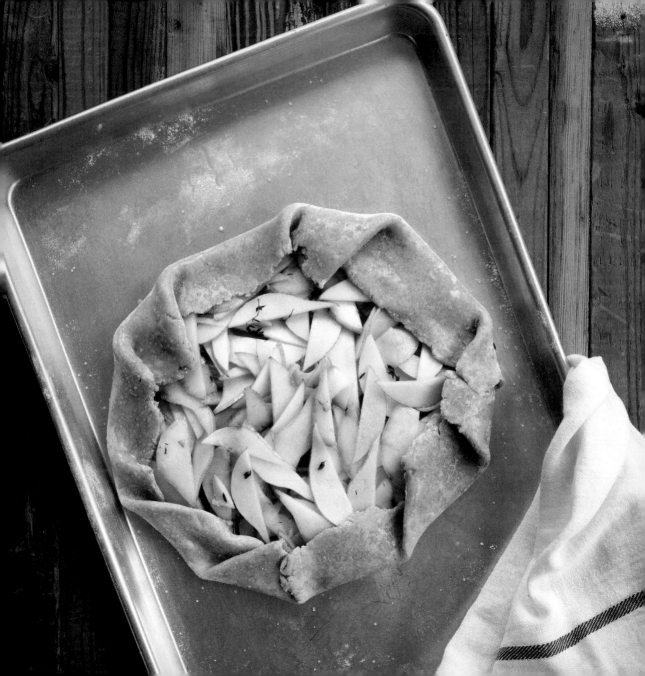

DESSERTS

There are three types of dessert people in the world: the chocolate lovers, the fruit tart / pie / crumble enthusiasts, and the creamy stuff connoisseurs. This chapter has something for them all. I personally believe that two desserts are better than one (I'm sure your friends won't mind, either), so I recommend serving the galette with either the chocolate bark or the *panna cotta*, which is totally doable, since the latter two can be made a day in advance. Of course, feel free to just serve one, too—all these desserts go well with all the menus.

Pear-Thyme Whole Wheat Galette
91

Vegan Autumn-Spice Panna Cotta
93

Spicy Dark Chocolate Bark with Cranberries, Hazelnuts, and Sea Salt
96

NOTE
Both the chocolate bark and the panna cotta are vegan and gluten-free.

A LITTLE HELP FROM YOUR FRIENDS
We all have a wine snob in our friend group, amiright? Ask him or her to bring a grown-up digestif, like sherry or port. Another idea is, well, more dessert: ice cream, candy, pastries from a local bakery . . . It's the holidays—live a little!

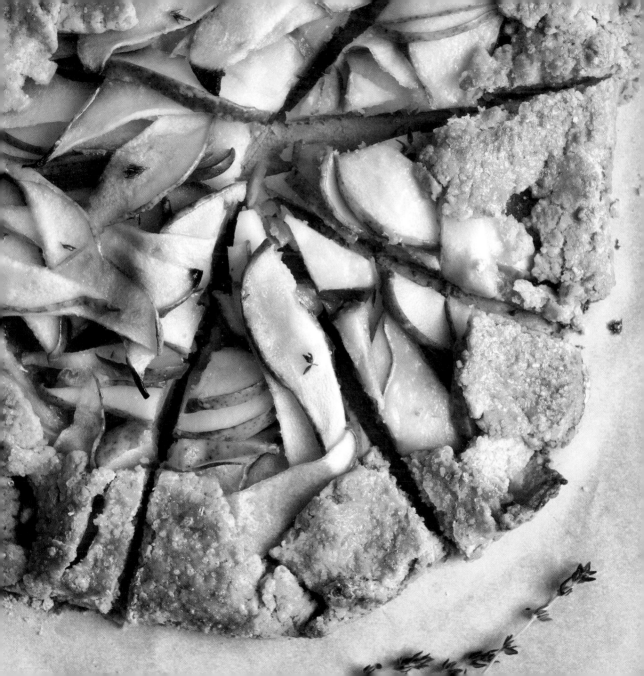

PEAR-THYME WHOLE WHEAT GALETTE

Making your own pie crust can seem intimidating, but there's really nothing to fear as long as you keep a few rules in mind. The main goal is to end up with a flaky crust, which is easy to achieve with these few rules: (1) Use really, really cold butter, (2) Do not overwork the dough, and (3) Keep the dough cold the whole time until the moment it goes into the oven.

CRUST

1½ cups whole wheat pastry flour, plus more for dusting (see Note, page 92)

1 teaspoon sugar

½ teaspoon fine sea salt

9 tablespoons cold unsalted butter, cut into cubes (see Note, page 92)

About ⅓ cup ice water

FILLING AND ASSEMBLY

2 ripe Bartlett pears (about 1 pound), cored and very thinly sliced

2 fresh thyme sprigs, leaves picked (about 1 teaspoon)

continues on next page

1. Make the crust: In a food processor fitted with the blade attachment, combine the flour, sugar, and salt and pulse to combine. Add the butter and pulse 10 to 12 times, until the butter turns into pea-size pieces (don't worry if the pieces are not all the same size). With the motor running, slowly stream in the ice water, just until the dough comes together against the side of the food processor.

2. Turn out the dough onto a lightly floured surface and gently knead it once or twice to gather it into a disk—do not overwork the dough. Wrap in plastic and refrigerate for at least 1 hour or up to several days.

3. Preheat the oven to 400°F. Line a baking sheet with parchment paper and set aside. Remove the dough from the fridge and let it rest at room temperature for about 5 minutes.

4. Meanwhile, make the filling: Combine the pears, thyme, lemon juice, and 1 tablespoon of the sugar and toss to coat.

1 tablespoon freshly
squeezed lemon juice

2 tablespoons sugar

1 egg, beaten

1 tablespoon unsalted
butter, cut into small
pieces

1 pint vanilla ice cream, for
serving (optional)

5. Unwrap the dough, place it on a lightly floured surface, and roll it out into a 13- to 14-inch circle (don't worry about perfect edges, a galette is meant to be rustic). Transfer the dough onto the prepared baking sheet. Spread the pear mixture in the center of the dough, leaving a 2-inch border. Gently fold over the dough edges. Brush the edges with the egg and sprinkle with the remaining 1 tablespoon sugar. Crumble the butter over the pears.

6. Bake until the pears are lightly browned and the crust is golden, about 35 minutes. If the pears are starting to burn, loosely tent the center of the galette with foil.

7. Let the galette cool for 5 minutes before slicing. Enjoy warm and serve with vanilla ice cream (if using).

NOTE: *If you can't find whole wheat pastry flour in your local store, use equal parts all-purpose flour and whole wheat flour. To get the butter appropriately cold, I cube it and place it in the freezer for 5 to 10 minutes before mixing the dough.*

FRIENDSGIVING PRO TIP

If you're attending other Friendsgiving parties this season, this dessert travels really well—just be sure to buy a paper box from a local bakery to bring it in. Have a few minutes to spare to make this dessert extra special? Cut the dough out into eight individual circles or squares to make mini galettes! People go crazy for mini things.

VEGAN AUTUMN-SPICE PANNA COTTA

MAKES 8 SERVINGS

This dessert features rock-star ingredients like creamy coconut milk and agar (a vegan gelatin substitute derived from a sea vegetable) to make an indulgent dairy-free dessert that tastes like autumn in a glass.

Two 14-ounce cans unsweetened full-fat coconut milk (see Note, page 94)

½ cup filtered water

⅓ cup pure maple syrup

1 tablespoon agar flakes (see Note, page 94)

½ teaspoon ground cinnamon

½ teaspoon ground ginger

½ teaspoon ground cardamom

Pinch of freshly grated nutmeg

Pinch of sea salt

1 cup large unsweetened coconut flakes

1. Place the coconut milk, water, maple syrup, agar, cinnamon, ginger, cardamom, nutmeg, and sea salt in a medium pot and stir to combine. Let stand for 15 minutes.

2. Meanwhile, set 8 small serving glasses or bowls on a tray or baking sheet. Set aside.

3. Bring the coconut milk mixture to a bare simmer over medium heat, whisking occasionally to prevent the agar from sticking to the bottom. Reduce the heat to low and cook until the agar is completely dissolved and the mixture has thickened, whisking occasionally, about 10 minutes. To check if the agar has dissolved, tilt the pan forward to see the bottom—if you see flecks of agar, it is not yet dissolved. Let cool for about 5 minutes.

4. Divide the mixture among the prepared serving glasses and refrigerate (if a film has formed on the surface of the mixture, skim it off). After about 5 minutes, as soon as the mixture stops steaming, cover the glasses with plastic wrap. Continue refrigerating until the *panna cotta* is completely set, about 2 hours.

5. Meanwhile, preheat the oven to 350°F.

6. Place the coconut in a single layer on a baking sheet. Roast for about 5 minutes, until the coconut is golden brown; be sure to watch the coconut carefully, as it can burn quickly. Set aside.

7. Garnish the chilled *panna cotta* with the coconut right before serving.

NOTE: *Thai Kitchen brand of coconut milk—or another high-fat organic brand—is best here; steer clear of Goya brand, as it's too watery for this recipe. Agar can be found in most grocery stores these days—look for it in the Asian foods aisle. If not, find it in a specialty foods store or online.*

DO AHEAD: *The* panna cotta *can be made up to a day in advance and stored in the fridge.*

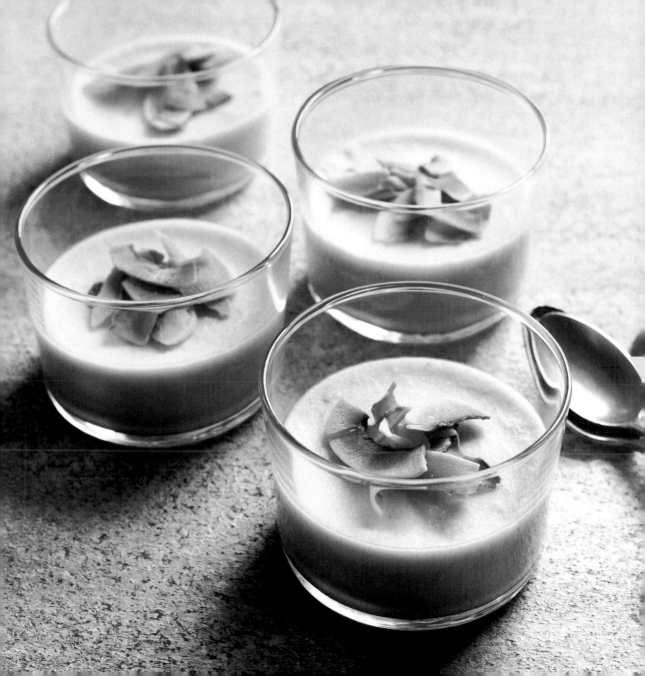

SPICY DARK CHOCOLATE BARK WITH CRANBERRIES, HAZELNUTS, AND SEA SALT

MAKES ABOUT TWENTY 2-INCH PIECES

Since this is such a simple treat, be sure to use the best-quality dark chocolate you can find (I love the Green & Black's brand). If you have vegan guests, make sure to use a vegan dark chocolate that does not contain whey or casein.

If you are wondering if you can skip the steaming method in step 3 and just microwave the chocolate, the answer is no. This French technique calls for a "bain-marie," or water bath, and involves gentle heating to prevent the chocolate from scorching and to keep it glossy and sexy. The microwave is likely to burn and dry out the chocolate.

Want to use other topping combinations? Try apricot, walnut, and sea salt; dehydrated strawberry; or pistachio and orange zest.

¾ cup raw hazelnuts

7 ounces dark chocolate, roughly chopped

½ cup dried cranberries or cherries

½ teaspoon coarse sea salt

¼ teaspoon ground cayenne pepper

1. Preheat the oven to 350°F.

2. Place the hazelnuts on a baking sheet and roast for 5 to 7 minutes, until golden brown and fragrant. Set aside to cool.

3. Meanwhile, bring about 2 inches of water to a simmer in a medium pot. Set a heat-proof bowl over the pot, making sure the water is not touching the bottom of the bowl. Place the chocolate into the bowl and let it melt slowly, stirring occasionally, keeping the water at a bare simmer.

4. Meanwhile, place the hazelnuts between 2 kitchen towels and roll them around under your palms to get the skins off; discard the skins. Roughly chop the hazelnuts.

5. Line a baking sheet with parchment paper and arrange the hazelnuts on it in a single layer. Pour the chocolate over the top. Chill for about 10 minutes, until it is slightly firm but still sticky. Sprinkle with the cranberries, salt, and cayenne. Continue chilling until completely set, 30 minutes to 1 hour.

6. Break the bark into pieces and serve.

DO AHEAD: *The bark can be made up to a day in advance and stored on the baking sheet, tightly covered with plastic wrap, in the fridge.*

 ## FRIENDSGIVING PRO TIP

Chocolate bark makes an impressive place setting/parting gift: place a few chunks into small decorative plastic bags, tie them with kitchen twine, and affix your guests' names to the bags.

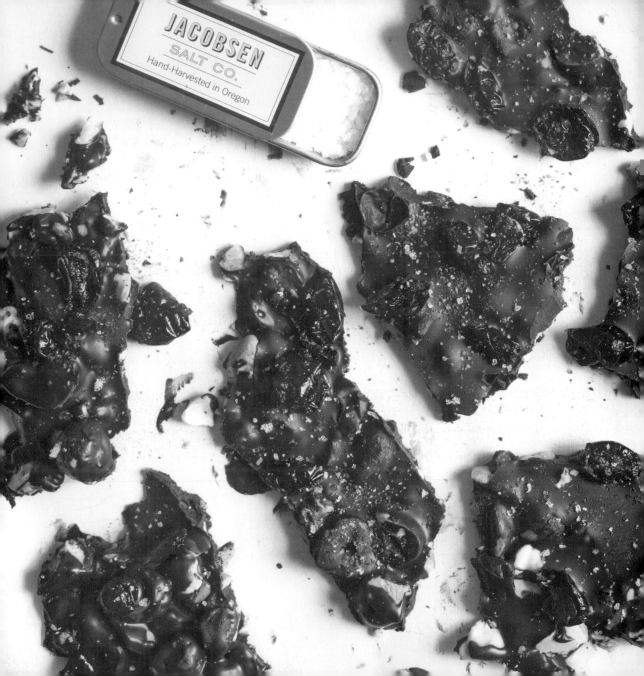

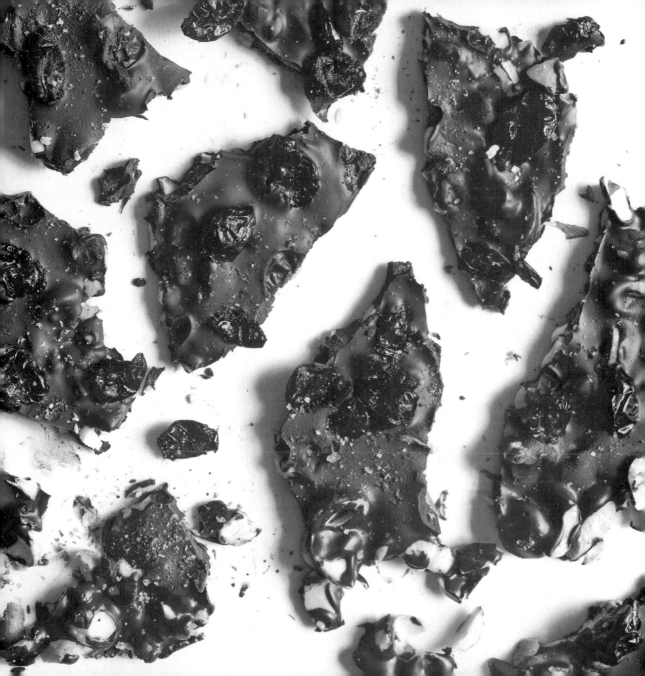

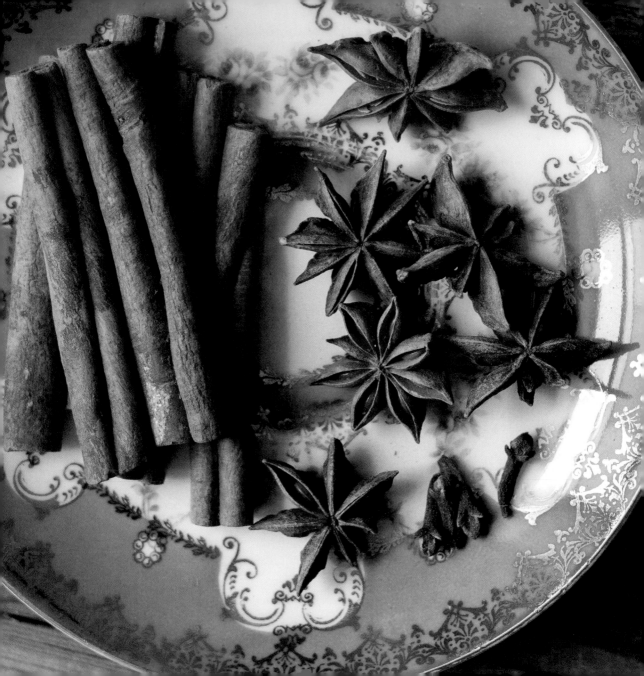

YOU AIN'T GOTTA GO HOME, BUT . . .

The dinner plates may be empty, but the party is still going strong. Keep your friends snacking and happy with a festive cheese board and warming spiced wine. Now you, the host, get to kick your feet up, too.

Cheese Board	Mulled Wine
103	104

A LITTLE HELP FROM YOUR FRIENDS

It's hard to go wrong with cheese board accompaniments like fancy crackers, a crusty baguette, cornichons, marinated artichokes, dried fruit, dark chocolate, stone fruit preserves (think plum and apricot) . . . the list goes on and on.

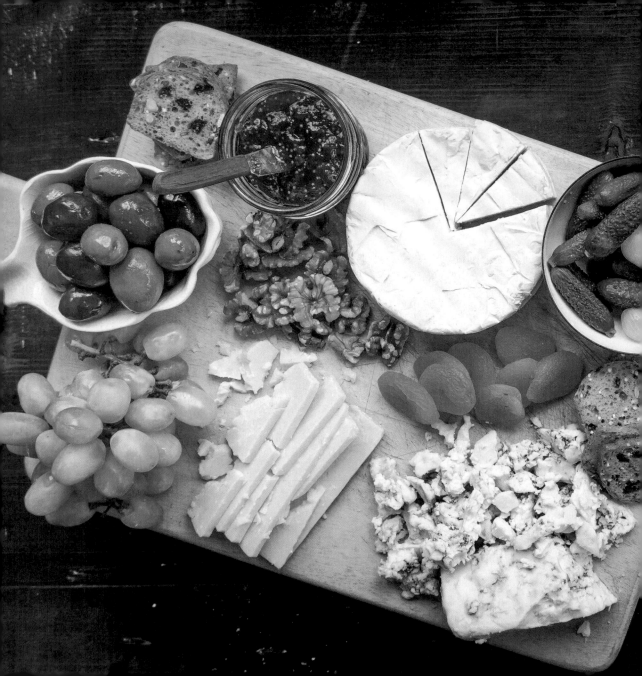

CHEESE BOARD

A cheese board is a beautiful and easy-to-assemble centerpiece for any party. The key to an irresistible spread is to have a balance of hard, soft, and juicy textures and sweet, savory, and sour flavors. Here's what to serve for a perfectly balanced board.

THE CHEESES

Three is the magic number. I always go with one creamy (like Brie), one hard (like Manchego), and one stinky (like Gorgonzola). Be sure to let the cheeses sit at room temperature, in their original wrappings, for at least 1 hour before serving.

SOMETHING STARCHY

Crackers (the cranberry-nut ones are perfect for Friendsgiving) and/or a sliced baguette.

SOMETHING ACIDIC

Cornichons, olives, and/or grapes.

SOMETHING CRUNCHY

I recommend walnuts, pistachios, or almonds, but almost any roasted nut will do.

SOMETHING SWEET

Dried fruit (like apricots, cranberries, or even bananas), a jam that's on the savory side (like fig), and/or honey.

MULLED WINE

Whether *vin chaud* in France, or *glögg* in Sweden, hot spiced wine is the official sign across many cultures that winter is here and it's time to slow down for a while. Remember those throw blankets I mentioned earlier (page 7)? It's time to break those out, too.

Two 750 mL bottles red wine
(see Note)

½ cup honey

4 strips fresh orange zest

Four ¼-inch-thick slices
peeled fresh ginger

4 cardamom pods

3 cloves

3 cinnamon sticks

2 star anise pods

1. Combine the wine and honey with all the aromatics in a large pot. Bring to a bare simmer (do not let the wine boil) and cook for about 10 minutes.

2. Strain, if desired, and serve in heat-proof glasses or mugs.

NOTE: *Choose a wine that you love to drink but not the priciest one of the bunch. The flavor will intensify as the wine warms, but it will also be enhanced with aromatics, so what you need is an in-between bottle. If you prefer not to buy all the spices individually, many retailers now carry spice mixes for mulled wine.*

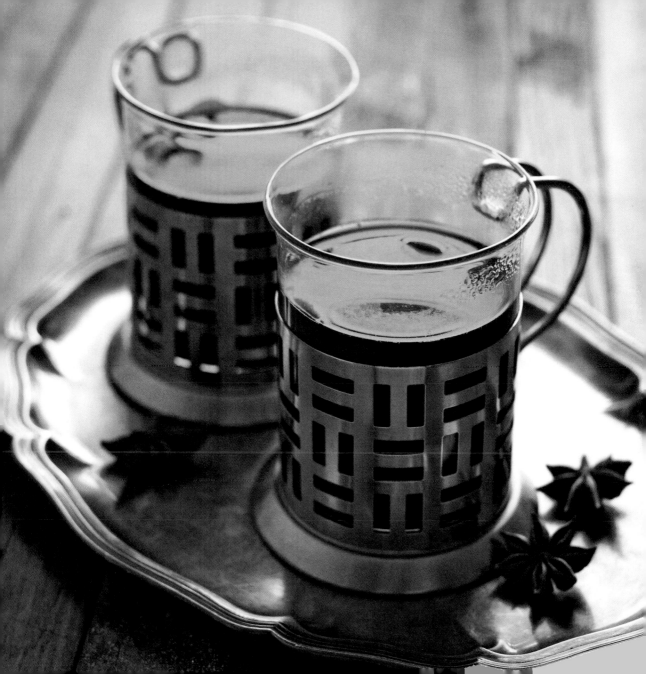

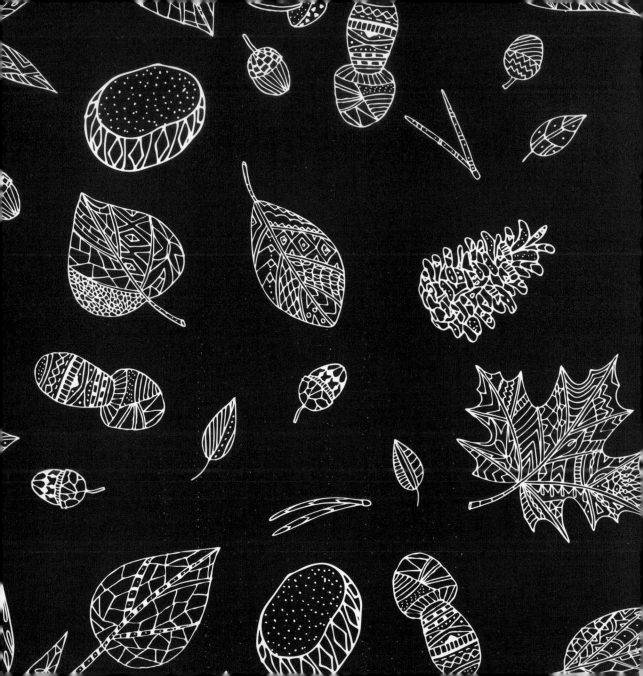

RESOURCES

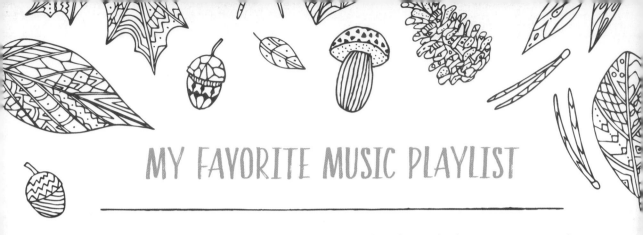

MY FAVORITE MUSIC PLAYLIST

A classy, thought-out playlist that sets the mood but doesn't overshadow conversation is the best way to elevate Friendsgiving or any dinner party. I like to keep it sophisticated (and on low volume) for the seated dinner portion using the playlist below. After that, I turn over the reins to Pandora for a Pink Martini, Gotan Project, or A Tribe Called Quest station.

"Blue Moon"
Billie Holiday

"Without Your Love"
Billie Holiday

"My Baby Just Cares for Me"
Nina Simone

"Let's Do It (Let's Fall in Love)"
Ella Fitzgerald

"They Can't Take That Away from Me"
Ella Fitzgerald & Louis Armstrong

"Almost Like Being in Love"
Nat King Cole

"I've Got You Under My Skin"
Frank Sinatra

"The Way You Look Tonight"
Frank Sinatra

"Stormy Weather"
Dinah Washington

"Beyond the Sea"
Bobby Darin

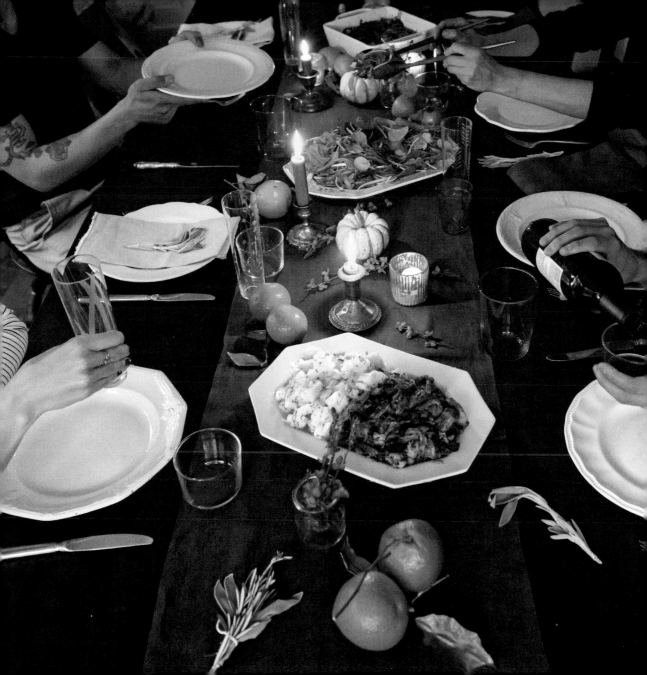

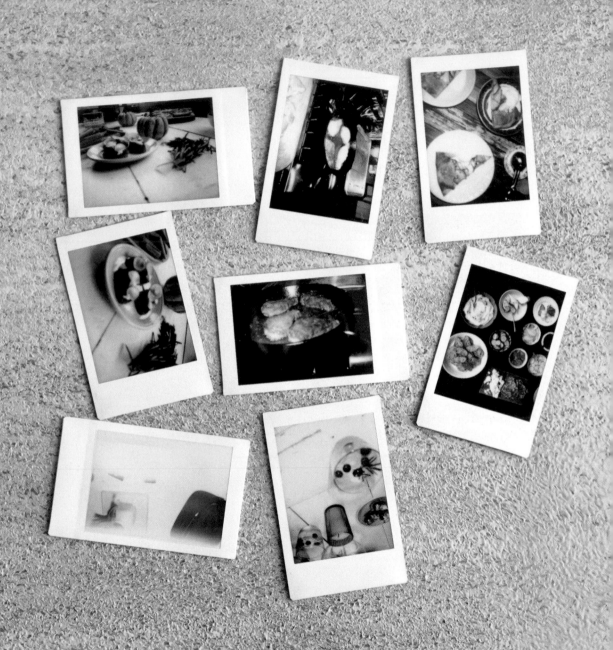

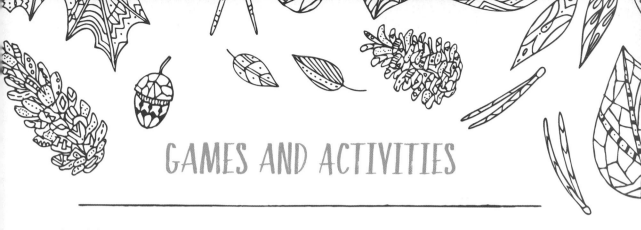

GAMES AND ACTIVITIES

Avoid the après-dinner food coma by playing some good old-fashioned games:

- ✎ Charades is always a riot. It's especially fun to play in girls-versus-boys teams.

- ✎ Fishbowl is another option—it's basically like charades on steroids, combining charades' miming with words and memory (look up the rules online).

- ✎ Card games like Taboo and Cards Against Humanity are also great to have on hand.

- ✎ There are plenty of party game apps for smartphones. My favorite is Heads Up!

- ✎ Having an Instax camera around is always fun. The mini instant photos make excellent party favors.

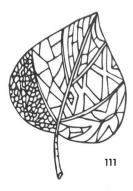

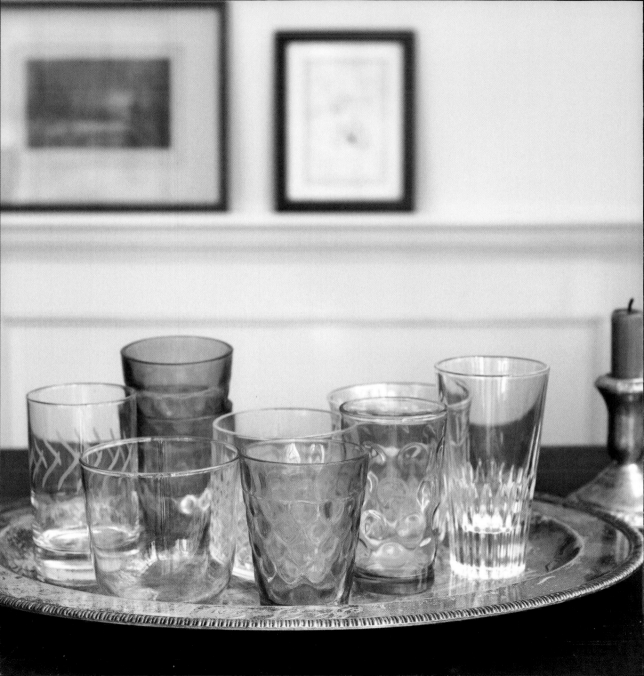

UNIVERSAL CONVERSION CHART

OVEN TEMPERATURE EQUIVALENTS

250°F = 120°C   350°F = 180°C   450°F = 230°C

275°F = 135°C   375°F = 190°C   475°F = 240°C

300°F = 150°C   400°F = 200°C   500°F = 260°C

325°F = 160°C   425°F = 220°C

MEASUREMENT EQUIVALENTS

Measurements should always be level unless directed otherwise.

⅛ teaspoon = 0.5 mL

¼ teaspoon = 1 mL

½ teaspoon = 2 mL

1 teaspoon = 5 mL

1 tablespoon = 3 teaspoons = ½ fluid ounce = 15 mL

2 tablespoons = ⅛ cup = 1 fluid ounce = 30 mL

4 tablespoons = ¼ cup = 2 fluid ounces = 60 mL

5⅓ tablespoons = ⅓ cup = 3 fluid ounces = 80 mL

8 tablespoons = ½ cup = 4 fluid ounces = 120 mL

10⅔ tablespoons = ⅔ cup = 5 fluid ounces = 160 mL

12 tablespoons = ¾ cup = 6 fluid ounces = 180 mL

16 tablespoons = 1 cup = 8 fluid ounces = 240 mL

RECIPE INDEX

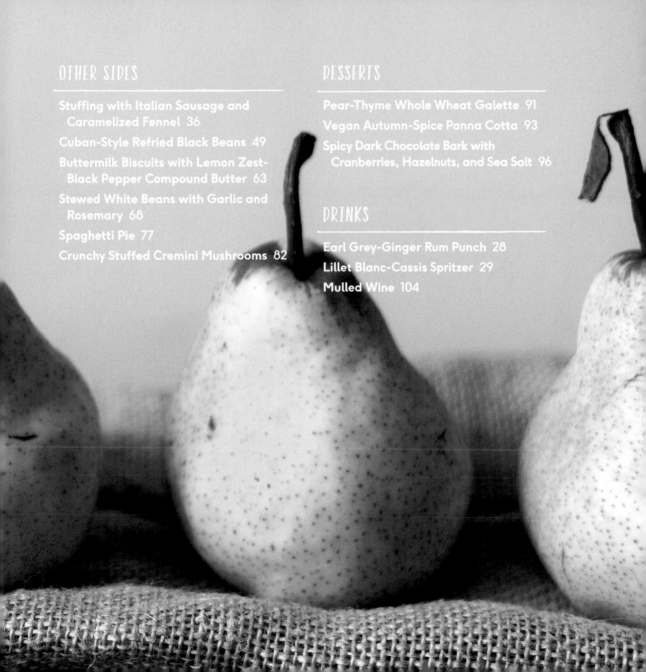

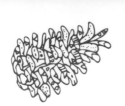

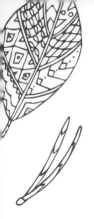
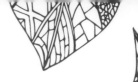

ACKNOWLEDGMENTS

Thank you to my editor, Kara Zauberman, for being the best collaborator a girl could dream of for her first solo cookbook. Thank you to my colleague and friend, Rebecca Ffrench, for providing support, many words of wisdom, and impeccable food-styling talents to this project. To my blog readers and everyone who has supported my endeavors throughout the years. To my boyfriend, Rene, for rooting for me, encouraging me to relentlessly pursue my dreams, and teaching me that everything is possible. To my sister, Lily, for being my loudest cheerleader and best friend, even if we don't get around to talking for weeks. Thank you to my friends, without whom Friendsgiving as I know it simply wouldn't exist. And lastly, thank you to my parents, who left everything they knew and loved behind to bring us to America, where dreams really do come true.

ABOUT THE AUTHOR

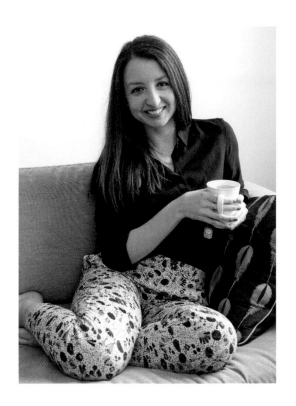

ALEXANDRA SHYTSMAN is a food writer and photographer, and the founder of *The New Baguette* blog. Her work has been featured in the New York *Daily News* and on Yahoo! Food, Refinery29, mindbodygreen, Gothamist, and ediblemanhattan.com. Born in Ukraine, Alex has lived in New York City since childhood.

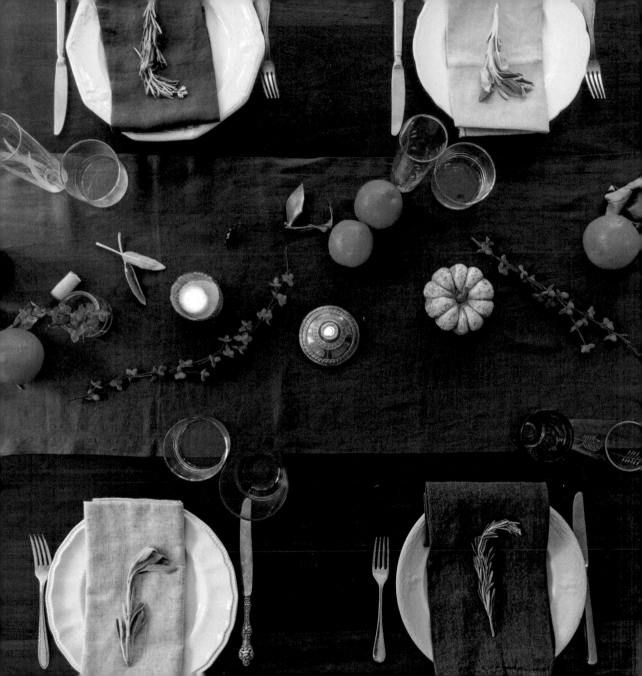